Health Policies in Interwar Europe

Research into public health policies and expert instruction has been oriented traditionally in the national context. There is a rich historiography that analyses the development of health policies and systems in various European and American countries during the first decades of the twentieth century. What is often ignored, however, is the study of the great many connections and circulations of knowledge, people, technologies, artefacts and practices during that period between countries. This book redresses that balance.

Josep L. Barona is Professor of the History of Science and leader of the research group Sanhisoc/Health in Society at the Universidad de Valencia, Spain.

Routledge Studies in the History of Science, Technology and Medicine
Edited by John Krige, Georgia Institute of Technology, Atlanta, USA

Health Policies in Interwar Europe

A Transnational Perspective

Josep L. Barona

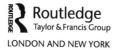

LONDON AND NEW YORK

First published 2019
by Routledge
2 Park Square, Milton Park, Abingdon, Oxon OX14 4RN

and by Routledge
52 Vanderbilt Avenue, New York, NY 10017

First issued in paperback 2020

Routledge is an imprint of the Taylor & Francis Group, an informa business

British Library Cataloguing in Publication Data
A catalogue record for this book is available from the British Library

Library of Congress Cataloging in Publication Data
A catalog record has been requested for this book

ISBN 13: 978-0-36-758792-5 (pbk)
ISBN 13: 978-0-8153-7091-8 (hbk)

Typeset in Times New Roman
by Swales & Willis Ltd, Exeter, Devon, UK

Contents

Acknowledgments

This book is a result of research conducted as part of a project entitled 'Health Policies in 20th century Europe', funded by the Spanish government during the period 2015–2017 (Ministerio de Economía e Innovación, MINECO, HAR2014-51859-C2-1-P). The author is most grateful to Jacques Oberson (League of Nations Archives, Palais des Nations, Geneva) and Lee R. Hiltzik, Assistant Director and Head of Donor Relations and Collection Development of the Rockefeller Archive Centre (Sleepy Hollow, New York) for their kind advice and collaboration in the management of archival documents.

I had the opportunity to discuss aspects of the book at the Bergen Workshops on Health and Medicine, organised by Astri Andresen, as well as during several panel sessions held as part of the European Social Science History Conference (Valencia, 2016) and European Conference for the History of Medicine and Health (Bucharest, 2017).

I am grateful to Josep Bernabeu (Universitat d'Alacant) and Kari Tove Elvbakken (University of Bergen), their comments and contributions when discussing the role of the national health institutes. Together with Bernabeu and Ximo Guillem (Universitat de València), I had the opportunity to address historiographical aspects and new trends in the history of public health. Some historiographical aspects benefited from discussions at the European University Institute (Florence) during my period as Salvador de Madariaga visiting fellow in 2015. Federico Romero and Laura Lee Downs gave me support and the opportunity to discuss viewpoints at this excellent international centre. I would like to thank Robert Langham, senior publisher for history at Routledge, and Julie Fitzsimons for their technical support and editorial comments. I want to thank John Rawlins for his support on linguistic revisions.

Abbreviations

ARA	American Relief Administration
DPH	Diploma in Public Health
IHB-RF	Rockefeller Foundation International Health Board
IHD-RF	Rockefeller Foundation International Health Division
IIA	International Institute of Agriculture
ILO	International Labour Office
INHA	Instituto Nacional de Higiene Alfonso XIII
LON	League of Nations
LONA	League of Nations Archives
LONHO	Health Organization of the League of Nations
LONHC	Health Committee of the League of Nations
LSHTM	London School of Hygiene and Tropical Medicine
NIPH	Norwegian Institute of Public Health
NKS	Norrske Kvinners Saniteitsforening
NIH	National Institute of Hygiene
OIHP	*Office Internationale d'Hygiène Publique*
RAC	Rockefeller Archive Center
RF	Rockefeller Foundation
SSI	Statens Serum Institut, Copenhagen
UNRRA	United Nations Relief and Rehabilitation Agency
USA	United States of America
USSR	Union Soviet Socialist Republics
WWII	World War II

1 Health policies in the twentieth century

A transnational issue

Why transnational history?

Historical research has traditionally been focussed from the perspective of nations and regions. This national perspective is especially overwhelming in political, social, demographic history; but it has also determined most of the economic, cultural, and scientific historiography. It seems natural that this is so if we consider that political decisions, as well as economic organisations and institutions, mostly depend on national structures and traditions, in other words, on the way nations are settled and organised. Identities, institutions, and values have been shaped in contemporary societies in accordance with national models. However, social, political, and cultural dynamics cannot be understood, and therefore explained, exclusively as the consequence of national patterns and internal dynamics. In modern times, it seems obvious that national communities are not isolated realities. International movements (such as the international public health movement) as well as expert groups, research networks, and international companies increasingly influence decisions, attitudes, and values. Non-national, external, transnational participants and agencies, often serve as references for emulating and legitimising national decision making. By giving most relevance to this perspective, a historiographical turn during the last two decades has stressed the historical importance of global and transnational history. A more global approach has been stressed for transnational actors such as migration groups, colonies, organisations, and professional associations.

Transnational history has also produced fruitful contributions on issues such as colonial history, human rights, democracy and education. This book adopts a transnational point of view on health policies, expert networks, and experimental medical research during the interwar years. When dealing with certain social and cultural issues, comparative and international history – traditionally devoted to the study of the relationships and influences among states, professionals, artists, or social groups – has been increasingly reoriented towards a much more comprehensive transnational history.[1]

However, the concept of *transnational history* has neither an exact meaning, nor a universally accepted definition.[2] This ambiguity may enable a more plural and richer interpretation, and this has contributed to its successful spread over the last few years. Several prominent university departments and research institutions now exhibit the label of transnational history as a hallmark. This also explains its rapid and productive expansion over the last two decades in numerous academic traditions and historical disciplines. This may appear as a sort of *global turn* in the history of international health. The use of a new vocabulary – using code terms such as transnational, circulation, appropriation – enables us to distinguish these new perspectives from the social and institutional history of international health.

A transnational approach to health policies deals not only with connections, interactions and comparisons.[3] It should also consider entanglements, clashes, rejections, obstacles, rivalries, and differences. At specific moments when health problems reach dramatic heights and become of huge political concern, we should pay attention to the transformation of ideas and practices, the establishment of political priorities, and the circulation of knowledge and know-how in national, international, and global spheres.

Transnational history has achieved meaningful influence in a plurality of academic traditions. It is worth highlighting its strong impact upon the historiography of migration, and colonial and postcolonial history. However, its influence on the history of science and medicine has been much smaller, and is particularly scarce for health policies. The history of public health remains dominated by the inertia of national narratives. I have tried to contribute a global and transnational perspective in my previous research on nutritional policies in times of crisis in my book on public health cooperation between the Rockefeller Foundation and the League of Nations.[4]

The lack of an agreement among historians on a precise definition of transnational history is not a meaningful handicap. Transnational historians stress the limits of national narratives and it serves as an alternative approach to the still dominant national perspective when dealing with the history of medicine. Nevertheless, the main controversial issues lay within transnational history's relationships to closely connected historiographical trends. Although, I do not consider it a fundamental issue, it remains difficult to distinguish transnational history from international history, diplomatic history, global history, post-colonial studies, or world history. Much of the difficulty revolves around academic discussions on occupying disputed territories.[5]

Transnational history could be partially understood as a crossroads, or as a meeting point, for different orientations that are trying to overcome the apparent narrowness of national perspectives. Furthermore, there is also a controversy on the plurality of non-national approaches and the primacy of one over others. The debate has a largely nominalist dimension. There is also a debate about whether transnational history is only possible when dealing with certain topics and specific historical periods. It is not my aim to enter into this debate. However, I am convinced that body politic, public health, as well as policies on hunger and nutrition, sexual and mental hygiene (among many contemporary medico-political interventions), can be better and more comprehensively understood from a transnational perspective.

Akira Iriye and Pierre-Yves Saunier, editors of the Palgrave Dictionary of Transnational History (2013), propose a relatively open and ambiguous definition. They claim that transnational history deals mainly with the links and flows, the 'people, ideas, products, processes and patterns that operate over, across, through, beyond, above, under, or in-between polities and societies'.[6] Despite being broad and ambiguous, this definition is eloquent as it highlights the fact that transnational history cannot be defined and restricted to a specific subject, nor a clearly shaped methodology, nor a corpus of knowledge. It is essential to understand that when talking of *transnational history* we are not referring to a historical theory or a research method. We are referring to 'an angle, a perspective',[7] that tries to establish a relationship between the historical topic of research and the position adopted by the historian. Consequently, this approach is the most relevant feature for transnational history, absolutely conditioned by the topics of research, and susceptible to be interpreted and discussed as links and flows, as mentioned above.

Other definitions of transnational history are not substantially different.[8] The Palgrave Dictionary assumes this open conception, and as it brings together more than 300 scholars representing a meaningful proportion of transnational historians, the consistency of the central idea is beyond doubt. At this point, it is worthwhile clarifying what is new in transnational history. Sometimes historiographical trends serve to re-conceptualise previous perspectives using a different language, and therefore it would be wrong to consider transnational history as a completely new approach to historiography. Much of transnational history could be considered as a further development of previous historiographical trends and contributions.

Connections between societies and nations have always caught the attention of historians, especially when dealing with diplomatic, political, cultural, social or economic history. The history of science and history of medicine is no exception. Science historiography has devoted research to the circulation of scientific knowledge and technology. The novelty of transnational history is the idea of offering an alternative approach to the dominance of a historiography structured around the nation as the main locus of scientific activity, technological innovation, healthcare policies, research programmes, and organisations.

Following K.K. Patel's metaphor, transnational history can be conceived as a manner of going beyond the *onion skin model*, where local, regional, and national history, on the one hand, and international and global history, on the other hand, are conceived as overlapping layers.[9] Transnational history defies this logic of layers by directly discussing national history as connected with local, supranational, or even global history. Transnational history provides tools and perspectives to go beyond the dominant principle of nation and territoriality in the organisation of historical facts (political, scientific or social).

When dealing with health policies, hygiene, healthcare, and experimental medicine, it is easy to assume that the health condition of the population, health policies, the gradual creation of the providential and welfare state during the first half of the twentieth century, necessarily involved transnational phenomena – and therefore cannot be fully appreciated and understood from a purely local or national perspective as if they were autonomous and self-sufficient. Sanitary campaigns, the fight against epidemics, research programmes to cope with social diseases, agreements about biological and pharmaceutical standards, healthcare institutions, preventive medicine, public health regulations, food quality control, and many other aspects related to health, disease, and medical practices cannot be related exclusively to national contexts. An understanding requires a transnational approach to discover the role of the participants intervening to produce the final results.

International relations and movements before World War One offer wide evidence of how links and flows can change, given that many of the ties were cut during the two World Wars and the deep social and economic crisis. Europe is a good example of a space endowed with strong transnational ties and, at the same time, a reality grounded on the strength of those bonds. According to K.K. Patel, if we try to understand what essentially characterises the *European* beyond national identities, a transnational approach would show to what extent medical and scientific interactions are important components.[10] Consequently, he argues that only with a transnational approach can we identify correctly Europe's place in the world, at least from the limited perspective of European history.

American historiography has contributed widely to the debates. Transnational history, as defined and advocated by various authors, including David Thelen and Thomas Bender, is mainly concerned with the movement of peoples, ideas, technologies, and institutions across national boundaries.[11] From this perspective, transnational history can be seen as an excellent approach to the history of science, technology, and medicine when applied to the long period – since the emergence of nation states are essential references in world history, and more particularly, in the European context.

In 1998, a seminar on transnational history was held at the *Instituut voor Sociale Geschiedenis* [Institute for Social History], in Amsterdam. The event was organised by David Thelen, then editor of the *Journal of American History*. After the seminar, the journal published a special issue entitled: *The Nation and Beyond. Transnational Perspectives on United States History*.[12] At the same time, a series of lectures took place at La Pietra (Florence, Italy) on American historiography. This series of lectures resulted in the publication of a monograph entitled *Rethinking American History in A Global Age* (2002), edited by Thomas Bender. Both publications are considered as major contributions to transnational history, the latter becoming the standard introductory discussion of the new approach.[13]

Therefore, at the turn of the twenty-first century, transnational history had become controversial and strongly influential among historians. It was soon related to global history, world history, and comparative history, although it looked for its own historiographical and academic space. Transnational historians usually criticise global history as being close to the modernisation paradigm (which expresses the unidirectional views determined in Western perspectives). Global history has been often criticised as producing an effect of homogenisation across the world. Nevertheless, it is recognised that the global perspective should be part of transnational history – and such a historical view aims to become a broader space, encompassing global history, including transcultural and inter-cultural relations. Transcultural and transnational history were also concepts and definitions discussed at the above-mentioned La Pietra meeting. The majority of participants considered these expressions as too broad and vague. The idea of transnational history enabled scholars to recognise the importance of the nation as a locus of historical research, while, at the same time, contextualising its histori-cal meaning.

Furthermore, transnational historians usually distinguish their work from comparative history. Nevertheless, such historians often had to make clear that comparative history could complement transnational approaches, even though they were not identical. According to the new viewpoint, historians must be aware that national spaces, institutions, and traditions change over time. Therefore, transnational history aims to put national realities in context and explain national dynamics in terms of its cross-national and supra-national influences.

The idea of a historiographical trend called *transnational history* first appeared on the agenda as a specific research programme at the beginning of the 1990s. The concept was suggested by Akira Iriye in 1989, when he argued in favour of a discussion of internationalism, as well as nationalism.[14] He suggested the study of an explicitly *transnational cultural history* that could complement purely national views and narratives. The same idea was proposed by Ian Tyrrell in an article pub-lished in the *American Historical Review* (1991).[15] Although the historiographical debate and the research programme proposed at the time were relatively new, the term *transnational* had already been used before in historical and in socio-logical discourse. It was also used in political science, for example, to describe the activities of multinational corporations and international labour unions in the 1970s. Robert Keohane and Joseph Nye edited an interesting early example of this genre of understanding: *Transnational Relations and World Politics*.[16] This book focuses mainly on state institutions, without paying special attention to the influence of transnational movements and flows.

As a further testimony of the ambiguous definition of transnational history, some historians consider that most of the research located under the Annales School could be labelled as transnational history in a broad sense.[17] If it has not been strictly considered as transnational it is because it was mainly focussed on cultural history without any national scope or reference. Some transnational historians remind us that at the Oslo sessions of the International Congress of Historical Sciences, held in 1928, Marc Bloch's contribution dealt with a compar-ative approach, but also provided ideas close to modern transnationalism and thus showed how transnational and comparative perspectives could be compatible and even complementary.[18] In his defence of the contributions of comparative history, Bloch highlighted productive explanations in a thorough analysis of communi-ties that are both neighbouring and contemporary and so constantly interacting. The work of the Annales pioneered research on cross-cultural and regional his-tory, and was strongly influenced by geographical conceptions. The most famous and cited example is that of Fernand Braudel, whose prominent research on The

Mediterranean and the Mediterranean World in the Age of Phillip II (1949) joined geographical, economic, and demographic orientations.[19]

Even accepting the evidence that transnational is a broad and ambiguous concept, it seems to be narrower and less extensive than either the deterministic and unidirectional notion of globalisation, or the excessively general meaning of 'trans-border' (which may refer to any sort of border – geographical, political, cultural, intellectual, between nations, but also within nation states, rural and urban districts, and even municipalities). The orientation behind the transnational label is more precise. It aims to focus on the relationship between nations and all factors beyond the nation, considering that the nation-state itself is the result of a transnational production. The interwar years show a radical transformation of the European national cartography.

Consequently, the limits of the nation, its geographical dimension, demographic evolution, economic structure, or social change are strongly influenced by competitive neighbouring countries, international groups, corporations, experts, and international pressure. No nation can exist in isolation as a product of its own internal dynamics. National identities have been shaped in continuous interaction with other identities, including the transnational phenomena that influences on the nation as it is constructed. This transnational making of the nation through a variety of borders from immigration controls to health quarantine, to state projects of national memorialisation, have only occurred decisively in recent times. Transnational history has put under scrutiny the traditional conception of nation as something natural, permanent, unquestionable, and understandable in itself.[20]

In recent decades the *transnational turn* has probably been one of the most relevant new developments in historical disciplines. It has challenged the traditional assumption that the nation is the basic unit of historical analysis. In doing so, transnational history has opened new perspectives, new research projects, and has produced historical knowledge that has revised and opened debate on previous understandings. Broadly conceived, transnational history follows across national borders and communities the circulation of people, ideas, artefacts, and practices. In addition, it also involves empirical research in national archives and other places. A long list of historical sources store valuable material, including: private and public institutions; philanthropy and humanitarian associations; international agencies; and corporations. The creation and evolution of public and private international agencies constitute an excellent space for historical research.

The term *transnational* strictly refers to modern and contemporary history, when nations are clearly defined. Nevertheless, it has been also used to describe regional areas of the pre-modern and early-modern periods. This orientation has been followed by research projects focused on the Atlantic world, the Indian Ocean, and the medieval Mediterranean. The ultimate goal of transnational history aims to discuss and reshape historical narratives grounded on the nation, and question the most rigid pillars of any form of nationalist history. If social history rewrote historical narrative from the bottom up, transnational history aims to introduce a new perspective from the outside in.[21] By focussing attention on the networks, circuits, and flows that lead social forces and shaping discourses and practices that span nations and cultures, transnational history has questioned the foundations of national history. In some sense, it is an approach that emphasises the broader context to deflate claims of national greatness and show that histories are more connected to the rest of the world and more in line with modern and contemporary societies.[22]

Circulating science and technology

This book adopts the perspective of transnational history instead of dealing with more or less autonomous national traditions. It is about national institutions, international networks, and public health policies, something that is closely linked to the social and political use of scientific knowledge and technologies. Indeed, the book deals with processes of circulation, appropriation, institutionalisation, and social use. At the same time as the initial debates on transnational history, research into the circulation of knowledge began to acquire historiographical relevance. The issue became an outstanding locus of debate in the late-twentieth century, particularly in the domain of the history of science and medicine. Previous contributions – such as the widely influential, discussed and criticised *The Spread of Western Science*, by George Basalla (Science, 1967)[23] – have had a great impact. Indeed, an earthquake was generated within colonial studies, regarding the processes of dissemination of scientific knowledge in the periphery and associated practices.[24] Implicitly or explicitly, most of these research studies contributed to the consolidation of global history and the notion of globalisation, conceived in a very unidirectional perspective. It was accepted that circulation happens from the productive centre to a passively receptive periphery. The model postulated the existence of active centres producing scientific knowledge and technological innovation, whose products – ideas, artefacts, and practices – were supposedly spread to peripheral territories. This reception takes place in accordance with a more or less permeable receptivity associated with social, cultural, and ideological factors. The centre-periphery model involved a unidirectional view on the flow of knowledge, artefacts, and practices circulating from the apparent productive centres (or focal points of knowledge and technologies) to passive peripheries that are conceived basically as mere recipients of what is produced elsewhere. Basalla's model – later criticised due to its simple diffusionist representation – could be subdivided into three successive phases, although these phases cannot be assigned to particular time periods given that colonial empires did not develop uniformly.

According to Basalla's diffusionist approach, the first phase was characterised by the exploring expeditions of European scientists, who applied their established scientific research methods to investigate new territories. In this way, new knowledge emerged. This initial phase, characterised by scientific expeditions, has a geographical representation. Western countries and territories appear as central, while some regions were scientifically discovered and described by voyaging researchers in early modern times. However, it should be accepted that this process did not stop until the twentieth century. For example, Japan, Italy, France, or

Germany were expanding their imperial projects to many territories until World War Two. In addition to variations in the temporal perspective, the geographical centres of science production and transfer also changed.

Basalla described the second phase of scientific transfer as 'colonial science', considering the subordination of colonial peripheries to the European centre. During this phase, scientists and technicians acted in the service of the European colonial powers, and given that they had been trained in the European centres they mostly remained focussed towards the Eurocentric orientation. According to Basalla's views, alleged colonial science was structurally and organically dependent on European research centres, due to its intellectual, technical, and institutional inferiority. Nevertheless, colonial science could also contain elements of autonomous scientific traditions in an embryonic dimension.

The third and final phase described in Basalla's model expressed the emergence of a separate and independent scientific tradition in the periphery, which would itself become, with the passing of time, a scientific centre participating in reciprocal exchange processes with other centres. It is important to highlight the fact that reaching a degree of autonomy with the peripheral colonies does not imply escaping the influence of Western tradition. On the contrary, Basalla identified colonial scientific independence as the successful adoption of Western science in the colonial territories. For this to happen, he identified a series of conditions, such as overcoming cultural and religious obstacles and resistance to the scientific method, and the establishment of national research institutions. In his famous article on *The Spread of Western Science . . .* , Basalla discussed the prevalence of Confucianism in China as a main factor preventing the development of modern scientific tradition until the late nineteenth century.

Even considering its Western centrality, one of the main contributions of Basalla's model was the attempt to analyse science transfer within Western limits and contexts, as well as providing an understanding of global transfer processes. However, his proposal has become controversial in several aspects. Global history and the globalisation process appear to be identified as the expansion of Western science, culture, and values.

After Basalla's initial contribution, other authors such as Edward Shils – an American sociologist and former editor of the journal *Minerva*[25] – as well as Joseph Ben-David, developed and expanded the centre-periphery model with great success during the 1970s.[26] Diffusionism involved the idea that the production of scientific knowledge applies mainly to a few central scenarios, usually associated with the major Western scientific, economic, and political powers. Conversely, peripheries were seen as territories and communities assimilating and receiving. Therefore, the main interest in studying science in the periphery was the debate on the factors facilitating or blocking new ideas, artefacts, methods, and practices from the centre – or the reception channels. In short, peripheries were considered to be rather passive scientific territories. Early studies on the transfer of scientific knowledge were predominantly understood as a matter of production and reception, as an export of modern European science to other non-scientific cultures, settling a conceptual difference between the Western centre and the non-Western periphery. Therefore, Europe appears to be the political and economic metropolitan power, as well as the epistemic centre of the world and the hard nucleus of the science epistemic community.

The distinction established by diffusionist sociologists and historians of science and technology between an epistemic centre and a subaltern periphery also provided the basis for another controversial argument: the so-called civilising mission of European culture and Western science. This controversial view applied to the extent that the colonial powers claimed for themselves a civilising duty, in which the export of science, technology, and medicine assumed a central ideological role.[27]

Nevertheless, since the late 1970s the exclusive focus on Western science as the hegemonic centre and a superior system of knowledge has been problematized in several historiographical domains, particularly in the context of postcolonial history. One of the most influential contributions was Edward Said's *Orientalism* (1978), an essay discussing Western representations of peoples and societies in Africa, Asia, and the Middle East.[28] The wide scope of Said's scholarship established a landmark in the foundation of post-colonial cultural studies. It discussed the implications of these representations in relation with post-colonial periods.

According to Said, the representation of the Orient as a cognitive opposite to the Occident is a discursive instrument of power, which not only guarantees European hegemony over the Orient, but also works as an essential element for the self-affirmation of European superiority. According to Said's views, much of the Western representation of Islamic civilisation was an exercise in political hegemony and power legitimation, an exercise in the self-affirmation of the superiority of European culture and identity. As such it was far from being the objective exercise of intellectual enquiry as should be expected from the academic research of Eastern cultures. Consequently, orientalism unveiled an intellectual construct addressed to practical and cultural discrimination that was applied by European academics to non-European societies and peoples in order to establish European superiority and imperial domination.

The so-called post-colonial theory has put into debate the mechanisms of dominance displayed by Western powers and especially their forms of intellectual enquiry and production of knowledge in the academic, intellectual, and cultural spheres regarding decolonised countries. Said's essay concentrated upon the British and the French varieties of orientalism that supported their empires – as built upon profitable commercial enterprises dating from colonial times.

After considerable initial impact, the centre-periphery approach continued to be discussed during the 1980s and faced critical views. The opponents lacked, however, an alternative theory to explain the circulation of knowledge, artefacts, and practices. Theoretical developments, mainly derived from post-colonial history, have since led to another shift in historiographical perspective with increasing attention paid to indigenous forms of knowledge, as well as to the connections and interactions between indigenous knowledge and Western traditions. Proposals such as that of Roy MacLeod contributed a new concept: the *moving metropolis*.[29] In the same critical direction can be seen the contributions of Paolo Palladino[30] and Michael Worboys.[31] More recently, Kapil Raj,[32] among others, have joined a long list of authors who have contributed valuable research materials that have served to question the unidirectional flow of knowledge implicit in the traditional centre-periphery perspective. They all have rejected, in one way or another, the traditional idea of *passive reception*, and instead describe an *active appropriation* of knowledge, highlighting the relevance of mediating factors, as well as the role of hegemonic elites. As a result of these new orientations, historical research has put more emphasis on the journeys of scientists, the internationalisation of laboratories and national research institutions, the role of scientific networks and expert committees, and many forms of education and science popularisation. These topics, together with a renovated perspective of transnational history, have achieved special relevance in the last decade.

A new wave of debate on the circulation of knowledge became especially visible in the historiography of science after the publication of *Knowledge in Transit* by James Secord.[33] In this work, Secord describes the fundamental importance of the circulation of knowledge for the history of science. His article suggests that the narrative frameworks used by historians of science need to come to terms with diversity by understanding science as a form of communication. Therefore, he proposes the centrality of the processes of movement, translation, and transmission, which were at the beginning of the twenty-first century already emerging in studies of ethnography, technology, history of ideas or cultural habits. Secord's approach offers opportunities for crossing the boundaries of nation, historical period, and discipline and shows an integrative capacity to overcome local and national perspectives.[34] Encouraged by the influence of the sociology of scientific knowledge, Secord advocated a history of science that was focused on processes of circulation and transfer of ideas and artefacts at different levels.

The renewed interest in global, international, transnational, and comparative history has also contributed to debates on how the circulation of scientific knowledge takes place in different contexts. Some of the approaches have taken confluence into consideration with the ideals and interests of the elites who have managed the globalisation process and tend to consolidate hegemonic forms of dominance and power.

Many of the most relevant recent contributions to the sociology of knowledge – especially found in works by Zygmunt Bauman, Ulrich Beck, Michael Gibbons, Bruno Latour, Helga Nowotny, Dominique Pestre, Alain Touraine and others – have raised new forms of conceptualisation.[35] These authors, among others, have greatly influenced research on the history and sociology of science, giving a new and more dynamic historiographical perspective to the analysis of the circulation of knowledge and the study of powerful networks of scientists, technologists, governments, and corporations. The complexity of the circulation process does not only consist in analysing the agents involved in the production, circulation, mediation, and appropriation of knowledge, but also in unravelling the relationships of power, strategies of control, and domination developed by hegemonic groups. Moreover, this complexity also applies to the transformation of appropriated knowledge.

The civilising process and *homo hygienicus*

Health emerged as an important part of the political economy in liberal societies during the nineteenth century. It was also a powerful tool serving the civilising process, as defined by sociologist Norbert Elias.[36] In modern Western culture, behaviour associated with the body came to be strictly regulated through a type of civilising process, in which moral norms and external prohibitions became internalised, while violations occasioned social punishment, as well as shame in the transgressor and disgust in others.[37] From the perspective of Elias, the late nineteenth and early twentieth centuries appear as a crucial stage for the expansion of this new body culture, closely linked to hygienism. Some authors have called it biopolitics, understood as a wide programme for disciplining behaviour, especially by means of sanitary intervention in the effort to move workers and peasants along the cultural and social path from backwardness to civilisation.[38]

Health and living conditions offered doctors and politicians several arguments in favour of biopolitics, because hygiene appeared as the main expression of the civilising process. Health, along with education, became the principal fields for social action, with the growing assumption that only civilised people could attain the rights and benefits of citizenship: an important political issue in time of crisis, scarcity, and war.

The civilising process and the policies generated by it can also be interpreted as the background to what Alfons Labisch described as the social construction of the *homo hygienicus*.[39] This represents the hegemony of the ideals and values imposed by the urban bourgeoisie with the legitimation of scientific knowledge and experimental medicine. The civilising process and the making of the homo hygienicus were powerful tools in the hands of hegemonic powers[40] acting in the domain of biopolitics, as defined by Michel Foucault.[41] He described biopolitics as a social and political power over life in a wide sense. In the work of Foucault, biopolitics denotes the style of government that regulates human life by means of biopower, or the invasion of political power in all the private and public aspects of human life. Foucault first discussed the concept of biopolitics in his lecture series *Il faut défendre la société* given at the *Collège de France* (1976).[42] *Biopolitics* and biopower appear as manifestations of the power of the state, considered to be the representation and principal tool of hegemonic elites over both the physical and the political bodies of the population. Foucault described biopolitics as '*une technologie du pouvoir*' [a technology of power], born in the frame of liberalism, whose main purpose was to maximise profits and make the body the cornerstone of market economies. The idea could be applied to health standards, nutritional policies, campaigns against epidemics, alcoholism, venereal disease, or infant mortality.

This was therefore the base for a new political concept of citizenship and the spread of civil rights. Hunger, extreme poverty, avoidable disease, child health, infant and birth-related mortality, and the abandonment of children, created a universe of intolerable situations, and these situations were targeted by liberal *biopolitics* from the first decades of the twentieth century onwards.[43]

It is easy to understand that the construction and meaning of the notion of *citizenship* has not been exempt from controversy.[44] The sociologist T.H. Marshall defined a triple dimension of the concept in 1963.[45] One is the civil dimension, which includes traditional freedoms of speech and thought, as well as freedom of movement and assembly. A second dimension is political citizenship, based on the ability to participate in the election of the government and political bodies, where decisions are made and taken. Certainly, all varieties of parliamentary democracy articulate different options of political citizenship. The third and most problematic dimension is social and economic citizenship. This third dimension consists of the right to enjoy minimum standards of living and the necessary social protection. In Marshall's words: 'the right to a modicum of economic welfare and security to the right to share to the full in the social heritage and to live the life of a civilised being according to the standards prevailing in the society'.[46] This third dimension of citizenship involves social inclusion and welfare and is essential for the development of the welfare state.[47] Nevertheless, the limits and extent of the third dimension of social citizenship has been problematized since the initial proposal made by T.H. Marshall in 1963.

Regarding the civil dimension of health and its importance in the framework of the civilising process, a key question is the political implementation of Article 25 of the Universal Declaration of Human Rights (Geneva, 1948) stating that: 'Everyone has the right to a standard of living adequate for the health and well-being of himself and of his family, including food, clothing, housing and medical care and necessary social services, and the right to security in the event of unemployment, sickness, disability, widowhood, old age or other lack of livelihood in circumstances beyond his control. Motherhood and childhood are entitled to special care and assistance. All children, whether born in or out of wedlock, shall enjoy the same social protection.'[48]

It seems obvious that considering health as a human right makes this right inseparable from the notion of citizenship, but in this case, some comment about equality and inclusion is necessary. In his influential work, Marshall recognised that the Poor Law – considered in its different national versions – was universal. Nevertheless, the minimal social rights derived from the New Poor Law were detached from the status of citizenship, treating the claims of the poor, not as an integral part of the rights of citizenship, but as an alternative to them.[49] Stigma remained, and it led to the 'divorce of social rights from the status of citizenship'. Marshall argued that the Poor Law was a system of relief rooted not in contributions and contract by citizens equal in rights, but as membership of the community. Poor relief was available to all who needed it as a matter of compensatory citizen rights to avoid exclusion.[50]

However, Beveridge (1942) based the universality of healthcare on contributions, pointing to the widespread expansion of the insurance system. Marshall's discussion of legal aid considered the problem of combining social justice with market prices.[51] He considered it important that: 'rendering of the service should not be conditional on the ability to pay', but open to all, and used by the majority rather than merely by the poorer section of society.[52]

Marshall's analysis applies to the context of the Cold War. The situation during the interwar years was very different. Going beyond the purely economic and political perspective, whatever the viewpoint, the first half of the twentieth century represented, from a social stand, a critical, contradictory, and essential period in the development of social citizenship. This was therefore a key period for the consolidation of the concept of citizenship and the expansion of civil rights, and where hunger, extreme poverty, avoidable disease, child health, education, infant and birth-related mortality, and the abandonment of children created a universe of intolerable moral situations. Access to health became not only an implicit right, but also an argument for trade unions and demands by social reformers for political intervention by the state.[53]

That same period also set a milestone in the cultural scene as a key factor for innovation, modernity, and progress. The new bourgeois society accelerated urban culture and appreciated cosmopolitanism as a positive value versus the traditional way of life. A long list of world exhibitions was opened in major European cities, art avant-gardes and any art movement that broke away from former conceptions and rules was worshipped, and a new model of universal citizenship expanded. This was in contrast with the impoverished image of the rural world, one that was increasingly considered backward, non-hygienic and crude, that is to say, not very civilised, according to the urban bourgeoisie idea of civilisation.[54] Similar cultural constructions affected the viewpoints of the colonies and non-Western contexts.

It was amidst this complex historical climate that the providential state emerged as a fundamental regulatory element in conflict management, social intervention, and stabilisation policies. Bourgeois liberalism and democratic ideals had to be shifted from the early nineteenth century *laissez-faire* attitudes that detested the state, to active commitment, usually in the form of a protective or providential state. The state, as the main guarantor and defender of the common good, appeared as an unavoidable means for implementing human rights associated with new values and rights of citizenship. The state broke through as a regulator, controlling and regulating people's social lives to prevent abuse. It was legitimated as the guarantor of social wellbeing, regulating the economy, encouraging scientific activity, developing social care programmes, building hygienic housing, cities, clean schools, and designing new suburbs. During the interwar years, the state emerged as the regulator of inequalities and the main advocate of people's rights. Consequently, Western countries developed an increasingly strong public administration that dealt with social order, including healthcare, both locally and nationally. But local and national policies were closely determined by international powers, transnational movements, and expert networks.

In addition, the supra-national dimension of social, political, and economic problems derived from the consequences of the two World Wars and the Great Depression demanded the configuration of an international diplomacy (which was usually employed as a reference for state initiatives that regulated competition between countries and staked the boundaries of the most-favoured nation principle). During the interwar years, this international framework was focused on the League of Nations[55] to foster stabilisation policies on trade, the economy, and the main political conflicts, as well as to frame initiatives on international public health and promote *biopolitics* and *social medicine*.[56]

From a sanitary perspective, a new period started after various international health conferences and meetings on hygiene and demography, tuberculosis, cancer, infant mortality, vaccines, vitamins, and rural health. Via international organisations such as the International Health Board of the Rockefeller Foundation and the Red Cross, philanthropy became very relevant for international health in terms of stimulating cooperation between countries through networks of experts. Health problems affecting millions of people and associated with poverty and infectious disease could be challenged using experimental research and public health policies.[57] Individual rights, as well as social and political stability, were involved.

Relations between the various organisations involved in international and national health during the interwar years sometimes appear as cohesive forces creating a strong and dominant power. However, their relations were also problematic, provoking tensions, rivalry, and conflicts. This was the case between the *Office International d'Hygiène Publique*, the Health Organization of the League of Nations, and the Rockefeller Foundation.[58]

This book is the result of considerable research, which analyses how transnational powers established the conditions to dominate transnational *biopolitics*, preventive medicine, and public health. Therefore, it is mainly focused on European institutions although this not due to a Eurocentric approach. On the contrary: the book aims to unveil how Euro-American hegemonic powers influenced national policies, both in Europe, the colonies, and many other areas in the world. The interwar period (1919–1939) was important for Europe and outside Europe. Developments in the Americas and in European colonies were crucial for shaping health policies on the continent. North Americans and Latin Americans occupied leading positions in the *Office International d'Hygiène Publique* and in the Health Organization of the League of Nations, and supported the Pan American Sanitary Bureau created in 1902. In other publications, I have highlighted how international public health became a diplomatic issue.[59] The Rockefeller Foundation and the Health Organization of the League of Nations created international interchange programmes for public health experts. This helped create a wide international network. Moreover, the American government and American foundations had important programmes in China and Brazil, where similar learning experiences as in Europe were implemented. In our case, the European context serves as the field for discussion.

Notes

1 Iriye, A. *Global and Transnational History. The Past, Present and Future*, Basingstoke: Palgrave MacMillan, 2013.
2 Iriye, A.; Saunier, P.Y. (ed.) *The Palgrave Dictionary of Transnational History*, Basingstoke: Palgrave MacMillan, 2009.
3 Raj, K. 'Beyond Postcolonialism and Postpositivism: Circulation and the Global History of Science', *Isis*, 104 (2), 2013, pp. 337–347; Raj, K. 'Colonial Encounters and the Forging of New Knowledge and National Identities: Great Britain and India: 1760–1850', *Osiris*, 15 (1), 2000, pp. 119–134.

4 Barona Vilar, J.L. *The Rockefeller Foundation, Public Health and International Diplomacy*, London: Pickering and Chatto, 2015; Barona Vilar, J.L. *From Hunger to Malnutrition. The Political Economy of Scientific Knowledge in Europe, 1918–1960*, Frankfurt am Main: Peter Lang, 2012; Barona Vilar, J.L. 'Public Health Experts and Scientific Authority', In Andresen, A.; Hubbard, W.; Ryymin, T. (eds) *International and Local Approaches to Health and Health Care*, Oslo: Novus Press, 2010, pp. 31–48.

5 Patel, K.K. *Nach der Nationalfixiertheit: Perspektiven einer transnationalen Geschichte*, Berlin: Öffentliche Vorlesungen der Humboldt-Universität zu Berlin, 2004; Patel, KK. 'Transnational History', *European History online, 2010-12-03*.

6 Iriye and Saunier, *The Palgrave Dictionary* (2013), p. XVIII.

7 Ibidem.

8 Budde, G.; Conrad, S.; Janz, O. (eds) *Transnationale Geschichte: Themen, Tendenzen und Theorien*, Göttingen, Vandenhoeck & Ruprecht, 2006.

9 Patel, 'Nach der Nationalfixiertheit' (2004).

10 Patel, 'Transnational History' (2010).

11 Thelen, D. 'The Nation and Beyond: Transnational Perspectives on United States History', *Journal of American History*, 8 (6), 1999, pp. 965–975; Bender, Th. *A Nation Among Nations: America's Place in World History*, New York: Hill and Wang, 2006.

12 Thelen, 'The Nation and Beyond' (1999), p. 969–970.

13 Bender, Th. (ed.) *Rethinking American History in a Global Age.* Berkeley: University of California Press, 2002.

14 Iriye, A. 'The Internationalization of History', *American Historical Review*, 94 (1), 1989, pp. 1–10.

15 Tyrrell, I. 'American Exceptionalism in an Age of International History', *American Historical Review*, 96 (4), 1991, pp. 1031–1055.

16 Nye, J.S.; Keohane, R. 'Transnational Relations and World Politics', *International Organization*, 25 (3), 1971, pp. 329–349.

17 Tyrrell, 'American Exceptionalism' (1991), pp. 1037–1040.

18 Ibidem, pp. 1041.

19 Ibidem.

20 Ibidem.

21 Ngai, M.M. 'Promises and Perils of Transnational History', *Perspectives on History*, December, 2012.

22 Ibidem.

23 Basalla, G. 'The Spread of Western Science', *Science*, 156, 1967, pp. 111–122.

24 Ibidem, pp. 115–117.

25 Bulmer, M. 'Edward Shils, as a sociologist', *Minerva*, 34, (1), 1996, pp. 7–21.

26 Ben-David, J. *The Scientist's Role in Society. A comparative study*, Chicago: University of Chicago Press, 1971; Ben-David, J. *Centres of Learning: Britain, France, Germany, United States (Foundations of Higher Education) by Carnegie Commission on Higher Education*, New York: Piscataway-MacGraw-Hill, 1977; Ben-David, J. *Scientific Growth: Essays on the Social Organization and Ethos of Science* (California Studies in the History of Science). Edited by Gad Freudenthal, Berkeley: University of California Press, 1991.

27 Pyenson, L. *Civilizing Mission: Exact Sciences and French Overseas Expansion: 1830–1940*, Baltimore: The Johns Hopkins University Press, 1993; Pyenson, L. 'The Ideology of Western Rationality: History of Science and the European Civilizing Mission,' *Science & Education*, 2, 1993, pp. 329–343.

28 Said, E. *Orientalism*. London: Pantheon,1978.

29 MacLeod, R. 'On Visiting the "Moving Metropolis": Reflections on the Architecture of Imperial Science,' *Historical Records of Australian Science*, 5, 1980, pp. 1–16; MacLeod, R. (ed.) *Nature and Empire: Science and the Colonial Enterprise*, Chicago: Osiris, volume 15, 2000.

30 Palladino, P. 'Historical Perspectives on Science, Society and the Political'. In Pestre, D. (ed.) *Report to the Science, Economy and Society Directorate*, Bruxelles, European Commission, 2007, pp. 105–107.

31 Worboys, M. *Fractured States: Smallpox, Public Health and Vaccination Policy in British India*, Andhra Pradesh: Orient Longman, 2005; Palladino, P.; Worboys, M. 'Science and Imperialism,' *Isis*, 84 (1), 1993, pp. 91–102.

32 Raj, K. *Relocating Modern Science: Circulation and the Construction of Knowledge in South Asia and Europe, 1650–1900*, Basingstoke: Palgrave Macmillan, 2007; Raj, K. 'Colonial Encounters' (2000), pp. 130–134; Raj, K. 'Beyond Postcolonialism' (2013), pp. 340–347.

33 Secord, J. 'Knowledge in Transit,' *Isis*, 95, 2004, pp. 654–72.

34 Ibidem, pp. 654–656.

35 A selection of their principal works and contributions are included in the bibliography.

36 Elias, N. *Über den Prozeß der Zivilisation. Soziogenetische und psychogenetische Untersuchungen*, Basel: Verlag Haus zum Falken, 1939; Barnes, DS, *The Great Stink of Paris and the Nineteenth-Century Struggle against Filth and Germs*, Baltimore: The Johns Hopkins University Press, 2006.

37 Elias, 'Über den Prozeß der Zivilisation' (1939).

38 Barnes, D.S., *The Great Stink of Paris* (2006), pp. 20–21; Labisch, A. *Homo Hygienicus. Gesundheit und Medizin in der Neuzeit*, Frankfurt am Main: Campus, 1992.

39 Labisch, *Homo Hygienicus* (1992).

40 Gramsci, A. *Quaderni del carcere*, Roma: Einaudi, 1975.

41 Foucault, M. *Il Faut Défendre la Société*, Paris: Éditions du Seuil, 1997.

42 Ibidem.

43 Andresen, A.; Barona, J.L.; Cherry, S. (eds), *Making a New Countryside? Health Policies and Practices in European History c. 1860–1950*. Frankfurt am Main: PIE Peter Lang, 2010.

44 A general discussion is to be found at Oosterhuis, H. *Health and Citizenship. Political Cultures of Health in Modern Europe*, London & New York: Routledge, 2016.

45 Marshall, T.H. *Sociology at the Crossroads*, London: Heinemann, 1963.

46 Marshall, T.H. *Sociology at the Crossroads* (1963), p. 74.

47 Marshall, T.H. *The Right to Welfare*, London: Heinemann, 1981.

48 *Declaration of Human Rights*, Geneva: United Nations, 1948.

49 Marshall, *Sociology at the Crossroads* (1963), pp. 83–84.

50 Marshall, *Sociology at the Crossroads* (1963), pp. 124–125.

51 Marshall, *Sociology at the Crossroads* (1963), pp. 101–105.

52 Marshall, *The Right to Welfare* (1981).

53 Andresen, Barona, Cherry, *Making a New Countryside?* (2010), pp. 12–14.

54 Ibidem, pp. 15–20.

55 Weindling, P. 'Public health and political stabilisation: The Rockefeller Foundation in Central and Eastern Europe between the two world wars,' *Minerva*, 31, 1993, pp. 253–267.

56 Barona, *The Rockefeller Foundation* (2015); Weindling, P. (ed.), *International Health Organisations* (1995).

57 Breschi, M.; Pozzi, L. (eds) *The Determinants of Infant and Child Mortality in Past European Populations*, Udine: Società Italiana di Demografia Storica, 2004.

58 Palmer, S. *Launching Global Health: The Caribbean Odyssey of the Rockefeller Foundation*, Michigan: University of Michigan Press, 2010; Barona, *The Rockefeller Foundation*, (2015); Borowy, I. *Coming to Terms with World Health. The League of Nations Health Organisation 1921–1946*, Frankfurt am Main: Peter Lang, 2009; Weindling, *International Health Organisations* (1995).

59 Barona, *The Rockefeller Foundation* (2015).

2 Historical origins of health policies

From the last quarter of the nineteenth century until World War Two, most European nations experienced the spread of national hygiene institutions promoted by state administrations. These institutions were called on to implement social medicine and public health policies as the main coordinating body of state administrations in close relation with provincial and municipal institutions. The dimension and relevance of this historical fact requires a thorough analysis, which demands, as far as possible, a historical discussion and a proposal of explanation. Some of the national institutions have been considered from a national perspective. Nevertheless, due to its international dimension, this historical event requires a transnational approach.

To appreciate the dimension of the phenomenon, let's list those institutions and their dates of foundation: Instituto Nacional de la Vacuna (Madrid, 1871); Kaiserliches Gesundheitsamt (Berlin, 1876); Pasteur Institute (Paris, 1887); Königlich Preußische Institut für Infektionskrankheiten (Robert Koch Institute, Berlin, 1891 and 1901); British Institute of Preventive Medicine (Lister Institute, London, 1891); London School of Hygiene and Tropical Medicine (1899); Institute for Maritime and Tropical Diseases (Bernhard-Nocht-Institut für Tropenmedizin, Hamburg, 1900); Medical Research and Advisory Council (London, 1913); Public Health and Marine Hospital Service (Washington, 1903); Statens Serum Institute (Copenhagen, 1902); Statens Bakteriologiska Laboratorium (Stokholm, 1907); State Serum Laboratory (Oslo, 1911); Instituto Nacional de Higiene Alfonso XIII (Madrid, 1910); National Institute of Hygiene and Public Health (Warsaw, 1918); and other similar public health institutes and national schools of hygiene in Zagreb (1925), Belgrade (1924), Prague (1925), Budapest (1925), Bucharest (1925), and the Istituto Nazionale di Igiene (1934) in Rome.[1]

Why were all these public health institutes established in European countries in no more than a couple of decades? Did their establishment share similar strategies? How did they relate to each other: cooperation or competition? Were they founded with similar aims, characteristics, and dimensions? What were their similarities and differences? Several plausible hypotheses come immediately to mind, but their relevance and similarities should be submitted to debate by historical research, and also as a global phenomenon, since they were established at a time when epidemics and infectious diseases were very prominent and affected international trade and public health during a time of widespread urbanisation and migration.

These institutions may represent the political response of the liberal state, a simple stage in the development of public administration under liberal reformism, and once health and disease became recognised as important political issues. Moreover, national institutes of hygiene emerged at a time when bacteriology, serology, and experimental medicine opened huge expectations for challenging infectious disease, child mortality, and so on. What Erwin Ackerknecht named laboratory medicine[2] involved new spaces for the development of knowledge, as well as a dominant experimental approach to research on the signs and symptoms of disease. Public health experts, serologists, and bacteriologists became new and powerful actors in the new landscape. Was their power as emerging specialists a relevant factor in the establishment of hygiene institutes?

During the last part of the nineteenth century, the first national laboratories were established for the production of vaccine in most European countries. Cooperation and rivalry boosted the social and preventive role of those institutions. They contributed to the health of the nation, and subsequently to national pride and identity. They also became a source of income for the nation, and a motor for a new industry based on health technologies. Should we conclude that the spread of national institutions of hygiene was the result of a process of imitation and rivalry among national research groups and institutions? Should we understand this transnational phenomenon as a case of centre-periphery expansion, where prestigious and scientifically powerful nations and institutions spread their power and influence over peripheral countries? Indeed, national institutions of health contributed to the building of the nation and to the expansion of public health, but also made scientific and technical contributions to national economies and international competitiveness. Competition among bacteriological and serum institutes could also be seen as cooperation among countries. A first approach shows plenty of international cooperation in scientific research as well as competition for money and prestige in certain aspects.

All these factors played a role to a certain extent. National institutions of hygiene were the nuclei of crystallisation of research programmes in public health, as well as the coordination bodies for the implementation of sanitary campaigns. They became research laboratories for fighting infections. This was the institutional expression of what Bruno Latour called the pasteurisation of France,[3] a response to social demands that also created new social demands. These institutions reinforced the political and economic dimension of health and disease. Nevertheless, it is important to remember that national health institutions did not play the same role at the end of the nineteenth century as during the interwar years. These research and public health centres experienced changes in their organisation, purposes, and orientation. Therefore, it is relevant to distinguish several historical periods.

National archives offer a national perspective for the institutes of health in their political and scientific activities, structure, and research. But they also contain letters, agreements, articles, reports, and documents that reveal international relations and research collaborations with other national and private institutions. This present research is mainly based on sources held at the Archives of the League of Nations at the Palais des Nations (Geneva) and the Rockefeller Archive Centre (Sleepy Hollow, New York). The League of Nations Health Committee and Health Organization did much work coordinating national health policies during the interwar years. Similarly, the Rockefeller Foundation Health Board/Division played an essential role in the structure, orientation, and funding of new initiatives. The following pages aim to offer a historically consistent picture of the transnational dimensions.

From public health to social medicine: the political dimension of disease

At the end of the nineteenth century, the term Sozialstaat was used to describe the state involvement in social reforms visible in Bismarck's policies in Prussian Germany.[4] The idea of a social state or État-providence brings us to the modern concept of the welfare state, a consequence of the idea of universal citizenship,[5] something clearly distinguished from earlier forms of poverty relief. The process of transformation of the Sozialstaat, as it was conceived at the turn to the twentieth century, until the birth of the welfare state after World War Two, was a hard road, hindered by conflicts and permanent international crises during the first half of the twentieth century. Considered from the perspective of social policies, some historians have conceptualised this period as the emergence of a sort of providential state with laws on working conditions (especially for women and children), labour accidents, unemployment insurance, healthcare, pensions, nutritional policies, and sanitary campaigns.[6] If the idea of such a social state was originally shaped in Prussian Germany, the development and expansion of the providential state had an international scope due to the huge dimension of epidemics, conflicts, wars, and unemployment that were always beyond the state's capacity for intervention. Most social policies implemented by governments, and particularly those regarding health, had a transnational background.

This research aims to analyse how national health policies were conceived and shaped under the influence of international networks of experts and transnational organisations closely linked to national medical and political elites and governments. Social medicine demanded scientific arguments, international legitimation, national institutions, and political decisions. Several approaches are possible when dealing with the issue. One perspective focussed on the social action initiated to fight certain diseases and conditions: tuberculosis; cholera; syphilis; hunger; and child mortality. Other approaches focussed on sanitary campaigns against high mortality rates, the implementation of preventive vaccination, and action against hunger and nutritional deficiencies. Although most of these aspects are present in the following pages, this book is mainly focused on the institutional dimension, and how expert networks and national and international institutions related to each other and operated. The importance of these efforts justifies a discussion on their connections and ideology, as well as how hegemonic groups gave technical advice that laid the ground for national policies.

Despite the fact that health and disease have always had important economic and political repercussions, public concern about health and disease did not reach a political dimension until after the end of the eighteenth century. The end of the *Ancien Régime* opened a period when authorities realised the importance of a healthy population for the wealth of the nation – and similarly the profound damage caused by plagues, infectious diseases, and huge mortality rates, especially when affecting children. Considered as an economic and social factor for stability, wealth, and conflict, health policies reached national dimensions. The popular and anonymous *Onania* (1710),[7] as well as the famous Samuel Tissot's *Onanisme* (1761)[8] – both translated into many languages and widely read all over Europe – not only moralised about the negative effects of non-reproductive sexual practices, but also tended to support policies to promote the growth of the population for the wealth of nations. Non-reproductive sexuality was viewed as an obstacle, together with epidemics, high mortality rates, and the spread of contagious diseases. Disease hindered the growth of the population and reduced the workforce.

It is generally agreed that Johann Peter Frank's *System einer volstandigen medizinische Polizey* (1779) was crucial for the spread of the concept of medical police, and for the inclusion of health in political strategies during the Enlightenment.[9] Frank was a doctor to the Prince-Bishopric of Speyer and in 1795 was employed by the Austrian emperor to run the army sanitary service and administer the *Allgemeines Krankenhaus* (the principal hospital in Vienna). He realised that poverty and disease were closely linked.[10] The ideological and political changes that took place during the Enlightenment contributed decisively to a political concern for health, disease, and the body. In this regard, Michel Foucault proposed the idea of biopower.[11]

Just after the French Revolution, The *Déclaration des Droits de l'Homme* was the starting point for the establishment of a *Comité de Salubrité* (1790) in France for the evaluation and vigilance of the health of the people. One of the members of the committee, Louis René Villermé, published several reports on the social dimension of disease and discussed them at the *Académie de Medicine* and at the *Académie des Sciences Morales et Politiques* in Paris. He explored the appalling conditions in prisons and compared epidemiological records in various Paris districts, identifying diseases affecting local poor people and the features of moral and physical degradation in the working classes in reports that thus linked poverty, exclusion, living conditions, mortality, and disease. Poverty and disease were identified as a stigma causing diseases and physical deficiencies.[12]

But the birth of biopolitics, or social medicine, as a political reaction challenging the negative influence of poverty and disease, was not only a French issue. Edwin Chadwick and the British Sanitary Movement, inspired by Jeremy Bentham's utilitarianism, also emphasised the influence of social factors in the varying extension and distribution of disease among population groups. William Farr's *Vital Statistics* (1839) – included in McCulloch's remarkable work *A Statistical Account of the British Empire* – pushed in the same direction as Villermé in France and raised awareness of the sanitary problems affecting the lower classes and the importance of hunger, poverty, and poor hygienic conditions as pathogenic factors. If we look around European countries, we see that these initiatives constituted an important issue for liberal reforms. Health statistics were a major contribution, since epidemiological indicators and surveys on the health conditions of workers provided new concepts such as life expectancy, which served to compare nations and social groups, and helped to conceptualise factors influencing health impairment (1842).[13]

In a similar way, German policies based on cameralism – the German version of British mercantilism[14] – reshaped former *medizinische Polizei* programmes and, in the mid-nineteenth century, several *Länder* started sanitary reforms focused on the state organisation of public health services. A national ministry of health was created as early as 1871, later followed by the establishment of state health insurance (*Krankenkassen*) as an expression of Bismarckian measures to offset the growing influence of the *Sozial Demokratische Partei* among workers in the new Germany. Meanwhile, Rudolf Virchow who published *Die Medizinische Reform* in 1848 following a request by the Prussian government, concluded that the most serious diseases were associated with social impairment, and therefore medical action had to be closely linked to political action. A view synthesised in his famous sentence: *Politik ist Medizin im Großen* (politics is medicine on a large scale). Other events and actors added new materials and arguments which reinforced the political dimension of health and disease during the second half of the nineteenth century. Max von Pettenkofer's surveys on health economics in Bavaria – *Über die Wert der Gesundheit für eine Stadt* (1873) – outlined not only the social, but also the financial benefits of investing in health and sanitation.[15] Similar initiatives took place in most European countries. These initiatives were the expression of nineteenth century liberal reformism. Liberals in Spain proposed parliament several reforms and initiatives, which finally led to the implementation of a Poor Act, the *Ley de Beneficencia* (1854). Liberals such as Mateo Seoane went into exile in London, where they were actively in touch with the British sanitary movement. They initiated hygienism, a social ideology that strongly guided municipal reforms during the second half of the nineteenth century.[16] Thus, with the consolidation of the political space of public health, the evolution of the liberal state, when it transformed into a providential state, included health issues as part of the body politic.[17]

In addition, experimental medical research contributed new scientific and technical paradigms. The new microbiological theory of contagion opened the door to immunology and serology, which created new expectations for preventive medicine to combat epidemics and infections. Bacteriology, immunology, and serology, together with statistics, and an increasing number of surveys on the economic cost of disease, contributed to the association of contagion, dirtiness, contamination, and lack of hygiene as a threat (sometimes associated with poverty, rural life, and unhygienic and insufficiently civilised ways of life).[18]

This perspective was reinforced by the emergence of social Darwinism and doctrines of race and degeneration applied to workers suffering from syphilis, tuberculosis, and mental diseases. Medical topographies, international health conferences, underpinned this approach with reports focused on rural and colonial settlings, as well as surveys made by governments and social reformers.[19]

The birth of public health

Health policies, public health, and bacteriology were also applied in the colonies, as they were in urban slums and poor rural districts. The French case is telling: seven branches of the Parisian Pasteur Institute were established in the French colonies between 1891 and 1914 and an extensive network of national and provincial institutes of health were established all over Europe around the first decade of the twentieth century. In each country, urban and rural health officers, local and national administrators, took part in this biopolitical mission. Disinfection programmes, vaccination campaigns, bacteriological laboratories producing sera and antiseptic products, rural healthcare centres, all show how public health was linked with scientific progress as a political tool for the conquest of poverty and squalor by means of experimental medicine. By the early twentieth century, health programmes and sanitary campaigns had become national policies throughout Europe.[20]

Around 1880, when the bacteriological doctrine of contagion became discussed and widely accepted, a key factor was added to the negative perceptions of the housing conditions of the urban and rural poor; the attempt to link squalor and unhygienic lifestyles with disease by means of the presence of a specific germ. The identifiability of each disease through the identification of specific germs as causal agents by means of laboratory techniques (serology and bacteriology) opened a new front in the battle against infectious diseases. However, the spread of the bacteriological approach did not necessarily contradict previous conceptions of contagion, as laboratory medicine often complemented the moralistic dimension of squalor and transgressions.

The late nineteenth century imperative of cleanliness was an important part of the civilising process, born as a social code reinforced by experimental science, so that public health concerns were strengthened and followed a more bacteriological laboratory orientation. The mutual influence of medical knowledge and moral principles played a central role in this sanitary-bacteriological synthesis. The recognition of germs as specific and identifiable causes added a qualitative difference to the traditional link between filth and disease. When pathogenic microbes were found in excrements, bodily excretions, contaminated water, infected food, and other substances, microbes became the main target of medico-political action. In some cases, rural districts were now depicted as unhygienic spaces endowed with a number of negative attributes: overcrowding; humans living under the same roof as animals; manure heaps; and uncontrolled defecation. To these arguments were often added a supposedly ignorant population, a defective and unbalanced diet, and high rates of alcohol consumption. In short, instead of the traditional romantically rustic portrait, the peasant's life became the archetype of unhealthy living and backwardness.[21]

The hegemonic hygienist ideology opposed the rural and colonial ways of life, where animals and manure were essential parts of the domestic economy and agricultural prosperity. With microbes directly verifiable through experimental methods, manure achieved pathogenic consistency, and was recognised as a health hazard as much as an agricultural resource. Yet the social ideology emerging around cleanliness also influenced peasant life and values. It is not easy to assess the attitudes of the peasantry, but there is evidence that people living in small rural communities had rising expectations regarding hygiene and cleanliness, not exclusively imposed by authoritarian hygienists, medical officers, the urban bourgeoisie, health administrators, and politicians.[22] Spanish rural districts were often a field for experimentation of new serological and bacteriological innovations without apparent opposition from the peasantry (who trusted the progress of science and accepted advice from the dominant elites). Professionals and experts were endowed with respect and prestige.[23]

International diplomacy and national institutions

International cooperation on public health started with a joining of forces to control communicable diseases. The first initiatives and agreements on health matters among national authorities were prompted by the need to protect trade by preventing the spread of cholera and yellow fever. From the central decades of the nineteenth century onwards, health occupied a relevant place in the international agenda.[24] The birth of what has been defined as an international sanitary movement led the way for national health policies to challenge the social consequences of disease. International networks and expert committees influenced the evolution of medical knowledge, clinical practice, public health policies, campaigns, and preventive initiatives in cities and rural districts. International health was a part of national diplomacy and played a prominent role in the international process of negotiation. This political concern also influenced the birth and expansion of a prestigious international scientific community that focussed on health and medicine and achieved growing importance in various domains. Its power was based on new forms of political and scientific legitimacy: negotiations of medical standards for biological products and pharmaceuticals; creation of national laboratories; expertise for institutes and public health schools; implementation of sanitary campaigns; establishment of international expert committees; organisation of international conferences on health and social issues (tuberculosis, venereal diseases, cholera, malaria, prostitution, nutrition, charities); and technical reports. Most practical uses of science and public policies were linked to the growing prestige and influence of expert opinions.[25]

During the second half of the nineteenth century, the main sites of experimental medicine and laboratory research were research institutes: these were either attached to universities or state administrations. These centres of bacteriological research (including vaccines and parasitology) offered technical advice on public health policies. They became a referential domain for scientists around the world – especially in Europe. Some American institutions, such as the Johns Hopkins

School of Public Health and the Rockefeller Institute, also played a leading role in the field. A wide range of young scientists began research in experimental physiology, serology, bacteriology, immunology, parasitology, and pharmacology – and thereby constituted a scientific international elite closely linked to governmental authorities. The research platform was based on a system of grants for young scholars.

Although the scientific importance of these research institutes did not decrease during the first decades of the twentieth century, after the end of World War One the internationalisation of medical science and the growth of international cooperation was led by two international organisations whose power of influence was exceptionally strong. One of these organisations was the International Health Board/Division of the Rockefeller Foundation, which established agreements with national authorities regarding public health expertise, funded sanitary campaigns, and offered grants, while aiming at creating an extensive network of well-connected public health professionals under its influence.[26] The other key actor was the Health Committee and the Health Organisation of the League of Nations, which prompted an ambitious international programme to expand public health worldwide by creating expert commissions, promoting international conferences, exchanging programmes and experiences among health officers from different countries, and promoting research and agreements in key fields. The committee gave a strong impulse to statistical studies and coordinated initiatives on diet and nutrition, drug consumption, rural hygiene, standardisation of biological products and pharmaceuticals, maternal and child health, and malaria. The strategy of improving the health of the European population was an essential part of international stabilisation policies at a time of huge social tensions, crisis, and conflicts.

Surveillance and control of epidemics had been a historical precedent of international intervention on health matters since central decades of the nineteenth century. Maritime transport was the key factor in disease transmission and local health committees applied isolation measures, quarantines, and sanitary cordons. The challenge of fighting cholera made national authorities of the most exposed countries – the Mediterranean coast and the Danube – establish unilateral systems of clean and unclean patents for maritime traffic. These regulations often allowed or restricted navigation depending on political interests and on the epidemic situation in the place of origin. It is unclear to what extent patents and quarantines were also used to interfere with trade for political and economic purposes. Indeed, after a terrible plague that affected Marseille in 1720 quarantine measures became increasingly rigid in maritime stations and involved the retention of ships for a quarantine period, disinfection of goods, and medical inspection of passengers.[27] The proliferation of these systems of patents and quarantine stations represent the oldest example of international health based on isolation from the threat, a model whose main goal was preserving cities and borders from the contagion of infections and disease from colonies or other infected places.

Feeling threatened by these national discretionary measures, which could damage commercial interests, European powers raised the need for international health regulations to address the spread of pandemics – but with minimum damage to trade. Diplomatic contacts between governments culminated in the celebration of a dozen international sanitary conferences, whose main result was the establishment of international regulations and sanitary stations for the implementation of rules to control infectious diseases. The Paris Conference (1851) was not the first attempt, and a long process of diplomatic initiatives had been underway since the early nineteenth century.[28]

To promote international agreements around quarantine regulations, the foreign policy of the colonial powers has traditionally been considered a fundamental factor. France and Great Britain tried to avoid protectionist policies that could harm their commercial interests. The rise of international trade during the first decades of the nineteenth century and the commercial interests of Western countries explained the support given to international sanitary conferences, in which diplomats, governmental authorities, and public health experts, met for discussion and negotiation. The sudden emergence of Asian cholera as a pandemic threat – scarcely known in Europe until the beginning of the nineteenth century – was added to the traditional epidemics and generated confusion at a crucial stage for colonial interests and the expansion of world trade. By the mid-nineteenth century, maritime trade had increased fivefold compared to the beginning of the century. The quarantine system and other restrictive measures implemented by states supposedly for public health reasons had become a political and diplomatic tool for the struggle between rival powers. In addition, epidemics were a risk for the health of the population and the sanitary control of ports and borders. The Vienna Conference (1815) opened a new stage of negotiation between national representatives, in which international conflicts became a matter of diplomacy and negotiation – rather than the use of weapons. A series of international conferences on health and demography, child protection, tuberculosis, milk depots, venereal diseases, and so on, gave way to discussions and agreements on specific issues, and these were much more effective in fighting the spread of diseases and reaching agreements on common policies. International sanitary conferences became a locus of intense diplomacy, whose interest extended beyond strictly health matters.

The establishment of quarantine to prevent the spread of epidemics and regulate trade from contaminated sites was an ancient practice that had been established in many Mediterranean countries since the mid-fifteenth century. Some cities had created local government bodies to manage quarantines. Preventive measures were usually applied to goods and passengers from the East, as this was the origin attributed to the plague, but ships from the West Indies were also controlled to prevent the spread of infections such as yellow fever. During the nineteenth century, the quarantine stations went through critical moments for political and commercial reasons, and health inspectors and authorities also discussed the extent of their usefulness. Trade problems caused companies associated with the import and export of products to pressure for change. Sanitary cordons along land borders were even less effective due to fraudulent schemes by traders to circumvent the law to protect their businesses. This controversial situation encouraged conflicts, criminality, and debate, and reinforced the idea that the key issue was to establish an effective system of reporting epidemic disease, rather than implementing isolation and quarantine schemes. But the establishment of an effective system of recording and reporting required international agreements, reliable and comparable recording systems, standardisation of diagnosis, as well as international coordination to ensure that reports issued by the ports of origin were reliable and equivalent. It was even more important that international epidemiological information was not handled according to purely political, military, or commercial interests.

This cluster of factors took the problem of epidemics into the agenda of international diplomacy from the end of the eighteenth century – at a time when the pressure from major trading companies against quarantines and sanitary cordons was increasing. Moreover, economic liberalism boosted international sanitary conferences to alleviate the tendency to state protectionism.[29]

Criticism of quarantines also incorporated scientific arguments against the new doctrine of microbe contagion that justified its application (associating the origin of the disease to the environmental conditions of the place where the contagious disease originated). The opinion of many doctors was critical to the effectiveness of quarantine. As a consequence, a series of studies on the conditions of occurrence of communicable diseases were carried out to highlight the importance of local sanitary and environmental conditions in transforming endemic diseases in certain regions into epidemics or even pandemics. Climatic and environmental determinism was conducive to this perspective.[30]

However, the explosive emergence of cholera in Europe during the 1830s caused a deterioration in the global health situation, amplified fears and hazards, and stressed the necessity for international agreements. The sense of vulnerability increased among the Europeans at a time when quarantine appeared as a means of isolating the infectious focus, and hence the only possible preventive mechanism. Nevertheless, ignorance about the causes and mechanisms of disease transmission and the controversial diversity of opinions left no room for unanimous further action. The first initiatives proposing an international regulation of quarantine occurred in the liberal France of Louis Philippe as an attempt to modify the previous Bourbon protectionism. F.E. Fodéré advocated convening an international conference in 1817 to promote agreements and regulations to end the chaos represented by the plurality of national quarantine legislations that lacked effectiveness and interfered with commercial relations.[31] Some years later, Nicolas Chervin (1833) again raised the issue in similar terms.[32]

The growing international concern about epidemics and controversy on quarantines opened the doors to diplomacy. In 1834, the doctor M. De Ségur-Dupeyron was commissioned by the French Ministry of Commerce to prepare a report on the various ways of implementing quarantine in Mediterranean ports. He made personal visits to the main harbours, studied their quarantines, and reported his conclusions to the minister. De Ségur-Dupeyron established a link between trade and epidemics, observing that there were no cases of epidemics in war areas where trade had been disrupted. He believed that preventive measures were necessary, but were ineffective as applied, and therefore recommended the establishment of a uniform system of preventive measures, ranging from short-term quarantine to the abolition of quarantine for ships from the West Indies. That strategy required, obviously, international agreements and despite the existence of an adverse climate for cooperation, in 1838 the French government hosted an international conference that gathered together representatives of European countries with Mediterranean ports to negotiate and agree a common system of quarantine. The proposal received support from two of the largest northern European powers: Great Britain (involved in major commercial interests in the Mediterranean in transit to the Middle East and India) and Austria (affected by numerous quarantine stations on both riverbanks of the Danube and along its borders with the Ottoman Empire). The participant powers aimed to generate international regulations and international conferences could alleviate the difficulties of international diplomacy and move towards a peaceful resolution of the political and commercial problems associated with hygiene.

The report produced by De Ségur-Dupeyron also influenced decisions affecting other Mediterranean areas and French colonies. A meeting held in Tangier in 1836, attended by Dupeyron himself, served to convene in April 1840 all the consuls of foreign states in Tangier to a meeting that was the starting point for the creation of a *Conseil Sanitaire Maritime International* [International Maritime Health Council] in the city. The strategy of surveillance and regulation led by France, Great Britain, and Austria spread to other southern Mediterranean zones such as Libya, Egypt, Ottoman Empire, and therefore similar international health councils were created in Tunisia (1835), Constantinople (1839), Alexandria (1843) and Tripoli.[33]

Although the 1848 revolution disrupted the work achieved in favour of international agreements around quarantine, France returned to the idea by proposing an international sanitary conference, which finally took place in Paris (1851–1852). Until the creation of the League of Nations in 1920, a long series of international conferences on sanitary matters were held in Europe and they became the most important open forum to discuss and negotiate international health regulations and public health issues. Negotiations and agreements implied more than just foreign policy, and various scientific concepts were also discussed, such as the latency period and the transmission mechanism.

The first international sanitary conference took place in Paris (1851) and relied on two delegates from each participating country: a diplomat and a medical expert. In his opening remarks, the French minister for foreign affairs noted the need to find a way of acting in accordance with technical and industrial progress, and called for international harmony through conferences and said the aim was to abolish the traditional political obstacles placed by local authorities and introduce free trade ports and borders. The participants were Austria, Sardinia, Sicily, Spain, the Papal States, France, Great Britain, Greece, Portugal, Russia, Tuscany and Turkey. But the conference can be considered a failure because the final agreement was only signed by France, Sardinia, and Portugal. The Mediterranean countries were reluctant to agree to the abolition, or even a drastic reduction in the quarantine system, while France and Great Britain pressured for minimisation of quarantines. The failure to establish an international agreement was due to a conflict of interest between the strategy of the economic powers to facilitate maritime trade and the still prevalent public health anxiety that called for controlling epidemics with quarantine and isolation.

A second sanitary conference was held in Constantinople (September, 1866) and was attended by 31 countries. France again took centre stage and called for steps 'to attack vigorously the Asian cholera in its original places . . .' rather than preventing its spread. The final agreements at the conference produced just a few resolutions on the expenditure of health patents by port authorities and healthcare control in harbours. As distrust predominated regarding the efficient management of quarantine stations, the possibility of stations administered by international joint councils was seen as an alternative. This option reinforced colonial power and generated controversy, as did debates about the duration of quarantine. The great commercial and colonial powers tried to put limits on the decision-making capacity of national authorities.

A third sanitary conference took place in Vienna (1874) and was attended by 44 representatives from 20 countries. Given the frustrating limitations of the Paris (1851, 1859) and Constantinople (1865) agreements, the Vienna Conference proposed a more drastic reduction of quarantine to benefit trade and thereby created tensions between those health authorities responsible for maritime health and border control in Mediterranean countries. The Vienna Conference established a distinction between land quarantine and maritime quarantine. In the first case only, each country was free to adopt the most appropriate isolation measures for sanitary cordons. However, maritime quarantines were a source of great controversy in the Caspian and Red Sea regions, and several European ports with a permanent medical inspection service approved disinfection and quarantine measures for seven days for infested ports and three to seven days for those under suspicion.

Sometime later, the Dresden Sanitary Conference (1893) convened diplomatic representation and public health delegates from Germany, Austria-Hungary, Belgium, Spain, Great Britain, Greece, Italy, Netherlands, Romania, Switzerland, and Denmark. Only diplomatic delegates from Montenegro, Portugal, Russia, Serbia and Sweden-Norway attended the meeting. The predominance of diplomatic representation over public health authorities was evident. The announcement of the conference convened by the Austro-Hungarian government established the main objective to be agreements that would prevent obstacles to the traffic of passengers and merchandises while providing uniformity to international measures. A reform of the Health Council of Constantinople was approved and an International Sanitary Board was created in Tehran, according to the reformed model of the International Sanitary Council in Egypt. International health surveillance stations were also established at the Persian frontier.

The International Sanitary Conference in Paris 1911 was the last milestone before the establishment of the League of Nations after World War One. Germany, the United States, Argentina, Austria-Hungary, Belgium, Bolivia, Brazil, Bulgaria, Chile, Colombia, Costa Rica, Cuba, Denmark, Ecuador, Spain,

France, Great Britain, Greece, Guatemala, Haiti, Honduras, Italy, Luxembourg, Mexico, Montenegro, Norway, Panama, Netherlands, Persia, Portugal, Romania, Russia, El Salvador, Serbia, Siam, Sweden, Switzerland, Turkey, Egypt, and Uruguay participated. An international sanitary convention that had been developing since 1903 was approved. Three technical commissions were established on yellow fever, plague, and cholera: each commission developing an agenda to discuss scientific aspects related to causes, transmission, incubation periods, symptoms, transport conditions for the contagion in maritime and land transport – and methods of prevention and disinfection.

Even if the international sanitary movement was closely associated with the emergence of cholera epidemics and quarantine as a political issue, other international social policies on health issues took place in the second half of the nineteenth century. At an international meeting held in Brussels in 1853 it was proposed to hold regular meetings with the participation of social policy makers in various countries. A couple of years later, in 1855, when the Universal Exhibition of Industry, Economy and Charitable Societies took place in Paris, the first International Conference on Charity also took place, and it was agreed to hold regular meetings to exchange experiences and initiatives to coordinate social policies. Topics included nurseries, asylums, host institutions for abandoned children, school hygiene, child labour regulations, charity kitchens, pensions for the elderly, care for the sensory deprived children, summer colonies, begging and child abandonment, charitable hospitals, and home social care. These events give an idea of the importance given to social problems during the second half of the nineteenth century.

These were the first initiatives for international meetings on *bienfaissance*, a French version of the German *Sozialstaat*, stressed by social policy makers in different European countries. The first *Congrès International de Bienfaissance* [International Welfare Conference] was held in Brussels in 1856, thanks to the initiative of M. Ducpétiaux, Inspector General of Prisons and Charitable Institutions in Belgium, under the auspices of the King of the Belgians, and the presidency of Charles Rogier. The minutes of the sessions and information about the various countries were gathered in a publication.[34] A second conference was held just a few months later in Frankfurt am Main. It received the support of German political institutions such as the Chamber of Deputies in Berlin. The organising committee was composed of politicians, lawyers, doctors, and priests. The *Congrès International de Bienfaissance* celebrated in Frankfurt was organised around three main areas: welfare, education and prison reform.[35] These welfare conferences show a growing expansion of international diplomacy around social affairs. The working programme was extensive and covered general aspects such as welfare, strategies to improve the working conditions of industrial workers, charitable institutions, public schools, domestic service, protection of poor children, child delinquency, alcoholism, compulsory education, childcare institutions, and the prison system. These conferences contributed an immense amount of information that circulated between countries, experts, and political authorities, and prompted the intervention of the liberal state in social medicine through active biopolitics.[36]

The third International Conference on Charities was held in London (1862), on the occasion of the Universal Exhibition together with a sixth meeting of the National Association for the Promotion of Social Science. The London conference was organised around two major topics: the role of the state in the fight against child abandonment; and universal education and compulsory school attendance. The following conference was held in Milan (1880), and in this case, the programme covered four areas: charitable organisations; charity by almsgiving; charity hospitals and healthcare; and charities and public policy. This last section included prisons and rehabilitation, as well as care for abandoned children, foundlings, and national legislative frameworks that referred to these issues. A novel aspect of the International Conference of Charities in Milan was the effort to encourage participating countries to report their national charitable model, the organisation of healthcare institutions, their operations, and legislative frameworks. Transnational networks were actively operating during the second half of the nineteenth century.

The *Congrès International de Bienfaissance* along with the International Conferences on Hygiene and Demography (1852–1912) and the International Sanitary Conferences were the driving force for national public and health policies during the second half of the nineteenth century. This was essential for the development of social statistics, public hygiene, and demography. The First International Conference on Statistics (Brussels, 1853) sought to discover the usefulness and application of statistics for the public administration in order to establish the foundation for a general international service. The initiative was raised at the Universal Exhibition on Industry (London, 1852). Immediately afterwards, a second conference took place in Brussels (1853), followed by others held in major European cities: Paris (1855), Vienna (1857), London (1860), Berlin (1863), Florence (1867), The Hague (1869), Saint Petersburg (1872), and Budapest (1876). The Budapest Conference focused on issues related to demographic and health statistics. Mortality tables were discussed and the main challenge was the application of international statistical methods to measure epidemics and assess public health.

Parallel to the celebration of the International Conferences of Statistics in 1876, successive International Conferences of Hygiene and Demography took place. Several meetings were convened in Brussels (1878, 1900), Paris (1880), Turin (1882), Geneva (1884), The Hague (1887), Vienna (1891), London (1894), Budapest (1898), Madrid (1907), Berlin (1907) and Washington (1912) and involved most European countries. At the turn of the century the seed was sown for international networks dealing with health politics and social matters.

At the International Conference of Hygiene and Demography held in Vienna (1891), the German hygienist Max von Pettenkofer, one of the active participants and promoters of sanitary conferences, spoke about the education of hygiene and preventive medicine in universities and medical schools. Pettenkofer was a convinced defender of the work done by the national institutes of hygiene in the implementation of experimental activities to develop testing and evaluation of sanitary interventions. While acknowledging the role of bacteriology, he highlighted that fighting infectious diseases depended more on government and social actions than on new therapeutic technologies. He thought that hygiene and public health should be taught at technical schools since there was a need to promote sanitary engineering, a key element in the prevention and resolution of many health problems. Many of the issues addressed in the International Conferences of Hygiene and Demography eventually became the subject of specialised conferences, as happened with the International Conferences on Occupational Diseases, International Medical Conferences of Work Accidents, and International Conferences for the Protection of Children.

The *Office Internationale d'Hygiène Publique* and the League of Nations

Throughout the preceding pages I have tried to offer a general overview of the huge amount of work achieved during the nineteenth century in the expansion of public health and international health. This is something not always recognised by current historiography when dealing with the national political response to social and medical issues. The importance and huge dynamism acquired by a wide range of international conferences and actors has been briefly summarised. All of these international events produced widespread networks, and created a strong impulse for the creation and circulation of hegemonic forms of knowledge which contributed to the implementation of new methods for social and medical research. This placed pressure on the authorities and governments in many aspects of social intervention on health and disease.

Nevertheless, the first institution officially dedicated to international health was the *Office Internationale d'Hygiène Publique* (Paris, 1907). The governments of Belgium, Brazil, Egypt, Spain, United States, France, Great Britain, British India, Italy, Russia, Serbia, Switzerland, and Tunisia signed in Rome, on 9 December 1907, an international convention for the creation of an International Office of Public Health, whose headquarters were established in Paris.[37] The governments of the Netherlands and Portugal also ratified the agreement – and a few months later Mexico joined the new international agency. The operating model consisted of a committee of government delegates whose powers were specified in an annex that included statutes for the office.[38]

The signatory countries were committed to participating in the operation of the office, which declared its independence from France and did not have to intervene in the management of health policies by member states. In the fourth article, the statutes declared: 'The office aims to collect and disseminate among the participant states facts and documents of general interest to the public health, especially with regard to infectious diseases, especially cholera, plagues and yellow fever, proposing measures to combat diseases.'[39]

Article 6 of the agreement attached to the statutes provided for the establishment of a permanent international board with a representative of each of the member countries. According to the statutes, the *Office International d'Hygiène Publique* inherited the interest and concern for international coordination in border health issues, a topic that had been often discussed in international health conferences. It exerted a permanent pressure on states to accomplish international agreements. Another main objective was the exchange of information on the general legislation and local regulations in different countries with relation to communicable diseases. The office showed interest in the impact of infectious diseases, public health statistics and epidemiologic records, sanitation projects, and other public health measures.

The office began its mission with courage by asking governments to send reports on the epidemiological situation of exotic infectious diseases, with particular reference to plague, cholera, and yellow fever, as well as the presence or breakdown of infections in colonial territories. Information was also requested regarding measures taken by national administrations to prevent the spread of these diseases. It seems evident that the international sanitary movement and the first national initiatives in Europe were the consequence of experimental bacteriology and the need to respond to hazards from the colonial territories. Moreover, the standing committee of the office requested information from governments about national sanitary legislation (laws, regulations, ordinances, decrees). The committee aimed to circulate this information, as well as reports on the general health organisation and the active public health campaigns in member countries, measures taken to fight communicable diseases, the organisation and operation of maritime health stations, and medical care in rural and urban areas.

The standing committee established a clear line of action with the international diffusion of public health policies in different countries. The *Bulletin de l'Office International d'Hygiène Publique* was a monthly publication that summarised this information. It was published in French and put political pressure on governments to regulate issues related to health and disease as a first step to implementing public health policies. During the following years, until the creation of the Health Committee and Health Organization by the League of Nations (1920), the bulletin became the main source of information regarding legislation and campaigns on statistics and epidemiological records. The bulletin reflected public health policies implemented by member countries regarding housing, slaughterhouses, sewage systems, and the control of the quality of drinking water to avoid the dissemination of infections. Epidemiological records on mortality caused by cholera, plague, and yellow fever worldwide were included in each issue, and this represented a real observatory for the prevention and fight against pandemics.

The *Office International d'Hygiène Publique* held two International Sanitary Conventions in 1912 and 1926 respectively, mostly focused on international regulations for epidemics and infectious diseases transmitted by maritime transport, quarantines, patents, sanitary passports, and migration as a vehicle for disease spread, mostly plague, yellow fever, cholera, typhus, and smallpox. The office tried to create an international framework coordinating public health regulations. In addition, it promoted a convention on anti-diphtheria serum (1930) and convened conferences on dengue and opium (1925, 1931). It also contributed to the coordination and improvement of national records and health statistics, and produced surveys on tuberculosis, venereal diseases, malaria, leprosy, cancer, typhoid fever, scarlet fever, meningitis, poliomyelitis, encephalitis, goitre, medical screening, rural and urban mortality, narcotics, drinking water, and hospitals.

When the Health Committee of the League of Nations was established in 1920, its president and several members of the committee were also members of the *Office Internationale d'Hygiène Publique*. Although it did not become a part of the League, the *Office Internationale* acted in close cooperation with the Health Organisation of the League, and in practice served as the general conference of the latter, i.e. it drew draft conventions, laid down general lines of policy, and so on. In short, it did in the domain of health much what the General Assembly did for the League as a whole.

On 2 May 1922, the head of the Health Organization of the League of Nations, the Polish bacteriologist Ludwik Rajchman issued to Wickliffe Rose, head of the International Health Board of the Rockefeller Foundation (IHB, RF) a report on Health Organisation activities since its creation in September 1921. He stated: 'A working agreement was arranged with the *Office Internationale d'Hygiène Publique*. Some 40 public health administrations from around the world are represented by governmental delegates on the permanent committee of this office . . . Its effective work has consisted so far mainly in the preparation of draft international sanitary conventions . . . The office however has no executive functions . . . and we are to be responsible for all executive work in the domain of international public health'.[40]

With these words, Rajchman expressed, in short, the project of a powerful international platform that would serve as a health policy authority for national governments. Who was to lead this platform? The policy of the organisation was formulated by the Health Committee, appointed by the Council of the League from among the members of the permanent committee, the *Office Internationale*, League of Red Cross Societies, and the International Labour Office (ILO). Scientific, administrative, political and geographical arguments were taken into account for the selections.

After World War One, the main participants in the network entered into action. The Danish serologist Thorvald Madsen was elected president of the Health Committee of the League and the Briton, George Buchanan, acted as vice-president. The Belgian, Oscar Velghe, was a member of the committee as chairman of the *Office Internationale*. Ludwik Rajchman was appointed head of the health organisation of the League. The Health Committee acted through the medical directorate and the health section served as the executive organ. As we shall see in the following pages, these new organisations in the frame of the League, together with the Rockefeller Foundation International Health Board/Division, achieved enormous influence in international and national health policies.

Notes

1 Since 1941 its name was Istituto Superiore di Sanità.
2 Ackerknecht, E.H. *A Short History of Medicine*, Baltimore: Johns Hopkins University Press, 1982.
3 Latour, B. *The Pasteurization of France*, Cambridge, MA: Harvard University Press, 1988.

4 Hüntelmann, A.C.; Vossen, J.; Czech, H. (ed.) *Gesundheit und Staat: Studien zur Geschichte der Gesundheitsämter in Deutschland, 1870–1950*, Husum: Matthiesen, 2006.

5 Habermas, J. *The Crisis of the European Union: A Response*, Malden, MA: Polity Press, 2012.

6 Pons, J.; Rodríguez, S. (eds) *Los orígenes del Estado del Bienestar en España, 1900–1945. Los seguros de accidentes, vejez, desempleo y enfermedad*, Zaragoza: Prensas Universitarias, 2011.

7 *Onania, or the Heinous Sin of Self-Pollution, And All Its Frightful Consequences, in both Sexes, Considere'd with Spiritual and Physical Advice to Those, who have already injur'd themselves by this abominable practice . . .* , London: H. Cooke, 1756.

8 Tissot, S.A. *L'Onanisme: Dissertation sur les Maladies Produites para la Masturbation*, Laussanne: Chez Marc Chapuis et Cie, 1761.

9 Frank J.P. *De Populorum Miseria: Morborum Genitrice*, Ticini: Delectus Opusculorum Medicorum; 1790. vol. IX, pp. 302–324.

10 Rosen, G. 'The Fate of the Concept of Medical Police', *Centaurus*, 5, 1957, pp. 97–113; Rosen G. 'Cameralism and the Concept of Medical Police', *Bulletin of the History and Medicine*, 27, 1953, pp. 21–42.

11 Foucault, M. *Il faut défendre la société*, Paris: Éditions du Seuil, 1997.

12 Rosen, G. 'Mercantilism and Health Policy in Eighteenth Century French Thought,' *Medical History*, 3, 1959, pp. 259–277.

13 Sigerist, H.E. 'From Bismarck to Beveridge. Developments and Trends in Social Security Legislation,' *Bulletin of the History of Medicine*, 13, 1943, pp. 365–388.

14 Rosen, G. 'Mercantilism and Health Policy' (1959), pp. 259–262.

15 Hüntelmann, Vossen, Czech (eds), *Gesundheit und Staat* (2006).

16 López Piñero, J.M. *Mateo Seoane, la introducción en España del sistema sanitario liberal, 1791–1870*, Madrid: Ministerio de Sanidad, 1984; Barona, J.L., Micó, J. (eds) *Salut i Malaltia en els Municipis Valencians*, Valencia: Seminari d'Estudis sobre la Ciència, 1996.

17 Rosen, G. 'Economic and Social Policy in the Development of Public Health. An Essay in Interpretation,' *Journal of the History of Medicine and Allied Sciences*, 8, 1953, pp. 406–430.

18 Labisch, A. *Homo Hygienicus. Gesundheit und Medizin in der Neuzeit*, Frankfurt am Main: Campus, 1992.

19 Barona Vilar, J.L.; Cherry, S. (eds) *Health and Medicine in Rural Europe (1850–1945)*, Valencia: Publicaciones de la Universidad de Valencia/Seminari d'Estudis sobre la Ciència, 2005.

20 Barona Vilar, J.L. The Rockefeller Foundation, Public Health and International Diplomacy, London: Pickering and Chatto, 2015.

21 Andresen, A.; Barona, J.L.; Cherry, S. (eds), *Making a New Countryside? Health Policies and Practices in European History c. 1860–1950*, Frankfurt am Main: PIE Peter Lang, 2010.

22 Baldwin, P. *Contagion and the State in Europe 1830–1930*, Cambridge: Cambridge University Press, 1999.

23 Barona Vilar, J.L. 'In the Name of Health. The *Instituto Nacional de Higiene Alfonso XIII* and laboratory campaigns in Spanish rural areas and African colonies, 1910–1924'. In Andresen, A.; Gronlie, T.; Hubbard, W.; Ryymin, T. (eds) *Health Care Systems and Medical Institutions*, Oslo: Novus Press, 2009, pp. 154–169.

24 Barona Vilar, J.L. Bernabeu-Mestre, J. *La Salud y el Estado. El Movimiento Sanitario Internacional y la Administración Española (1851–1945)*, Valencia: Publicaciones de la Universidad de Valencia, 2008.

25 Barona Vilar, J.L. 'Public Health Experts and Scientific Authority'. In Andresen, A.; Hubbard, W.; Ryymin, T. (eds) *International and Local Approaches to Health and Health Care*, Oslo: Novus Press, 2010, pp. 31–48.

26 Farley, J. *To Cast Out Disease. A History of the International Health Division of the Rockefeller Foundation (1913–1951)*, Oxford: Oxford University Press, 2004.

27 Bonastra Tolós, J. *Ciencia, sociedad y planificación territorial en la institución del lazareto*, Barcelona, Tesis Doctoral, Publicacions de la Universitat de Barcelona, 2006; Vidal Hernández, J.M. *El Llatzeret de Maó, una fortalesa sanitària*, Menorca, Institut, Menorquí d'Estudis, 2002.

28 Barona, Bernabeu, *La Salud y el Estado*, 2008, chapter 1; Harrison. M. 'Disease, diplomacy and international commerce: the origins of international sanitary regulation in the Nineteenth Century,' *Journal of Global History*, 1, 2006, pp. 197–217.

29 Ackerknecht, E.H. 'Anticontagionism between 1821 and 1867,' *Bulletin of the History of Medicine*, 22, 1948, pp. 562–593.

30 Livingstone, D.N. 'Changing Climate, Human Evolution, and the Revival of Environmental Determinism,' *Bulletin of the History of Medicine*, 86, 2012, pp. 564–595; Livingstone, D.N. *Putting Science in its Place: Geographies of Scientific Knowledge*, Chicago: University of Chicago Press, 2003.

31 Fodéré, FE. 'Lazaret'. In: *Dictionnaire Encyclopédique des Sciences Médicales*, Paris: G. Masson et P. Asselin, 1817.

32 San Martín, A. *La Conferencia Sanitaria Internacional de Dresde*, Madrid, Imprenta de Ricardo Rojas, 1883.

33 Barona, Bernabeu, *La Salud y el Estado*, 2008, pp. 25–30.

34 Two volumes were published in Brussels in 1856 under the title Compte rendu des debats du Congrès international de Bruxelles; session de 1856.

35 Congrès International de Bienfaissance de Francfort sur-le-Mein, Brussels, 1858.

36 Barona, *The Rockefeller Foundation* (2015), chapter 2.

37 Signatories of the charter were: E. Beco and O. Velghe (Belgium), E. de Salles Guerra and H. de Rocha Lima (Brazil), M. Tolosa Latour and P. Soler (Spain), A.M. Laughlin and R.S. Reynolds Hitt (United States), C. Barrère, J. de Cazotte, and E. Ronssin (France), T. Thomson and B. Franklin (United Kingdom), R. Santoliquido and A. Cotta (Italy), H. de Weede (Netherlands), M. de Cavalho e Vaconcellos (Portugal), Baron Korff (Russia), J.B. Pioda (Switzerland), I. Neguib and M.A. Ruffer (Egypt).

38 *Vingt-cinq ans d'activité de l'Office International d'Hygiène Publique, 1909–1933*, Paris, OIHP, 1933.

39 'Annexe. Status organique de l'Office International d'Hygiène Publique, Article 4', in *Vingt-cinq ans*, 1933.

40 Letter from L. Rajchman to Wickliffe Rose, Terrytown, New York: RAC RG 1.1, series 100, box 20, folder 165, 1922.

3 Networks of experts

National policies and transnational actors

The huge crisis caused by World War One and the subsequent Great Depression radically transformed the national cartography of Europe, as well as diplomatic relations.[1] Health problems directly linked to the deterioration in living conditions figured prominently among the most important challenges, and meant that governments and medical authorities had to cope with deep social crises affecting European countries during the first decades of the twentieth century. The challenge required a shift from the traditional public health control of plagues and infectious diseases – based on preventive measures such as quarantining and isolation – to social and preventive medicine founded mainly on epidemiology and health statistics, vaccination, preventive campaigns, nutritional policies, and bacteriological research.[2] The concept of social medicine emerged when society as a whole became considered as a living body suffering from social diseases, both infectious and degenerative, similarly to diseases affecting individuals. Empowered by state authorities, which sought to implement social hygiene strategies, social medicine tried to improve the health of the community and institutionalised a political and administrative apparatus to prevent and respond to social diseases such as tuberculosis, and venereal diseases, but also mother and child health issues, alcoholism, mental disorders, infections, hunger, and nutritional deficiencies. Social medicine was the central instrument for *biopolitical* strategies and the institutionalised response of the state to challenge the negative effects of disease on society.

Several important features were involved in this paradigmatic shift, one of which was the changing role of international organisations as they became technical centres of knowledge and expertise. The international context largely determined the orientation of medical research and also the patterns and orientation of national health policies, particularly in fields where international expert networks and committees appeared as endowed with technical legitimacy. In addition, international organisations and expert bodies played an important role in fundamental issues for the development of industrial science, such as the standardisation of research and clinical methods, agreements on the standardisation of pharmaceuticals and biological products (such as sera, vaccines, and hormones) and in instruction programmes for public health experts. These experts normally played a double role: they were part of international networks and they also belonged to national elites, closely linked to social medicine policies and decision making. They acquired growing scientific and political influence on public healthcare and in the implementation of health policies, inasmuch as they belonged to national and international advisory committees and expert networks endowed with scientific, technical, and political authority. Moreover, health itself became a prominent social and political issue during the first half of the twentieth century, as national constitutions started to consider health as an essential human right that should be politically implemented. Therefore, parliaments, public administrations, and the state itself emerged as dominant social regulators that acted in most liberal societies to palliate the negative effects of the crisis: hunger, unemployment, poverty, marginality, and the subsequent disease and social instability. For the liberal state, fighting for health was an unavoidable element of the wider programme to palliate the so-called *market failures* and social inequalities. It was the only way to mitigate the huge threat of social conflict and revolutions.[3] The growing influence of international networks and organisations on national health policies heightened the relevance of diplomatic debates and negotiations on implementing disease prevention and healthcare strategies.

Health and international diplomacy

The nineteenth century saw a gradual reshaping of the relations between nations. Following on from the Congress of Vienna in 1815, the Concert of Europe has been considered as a first attempt by diplomacy to organise the international sphere. It was an informal system of consultation between the Great European powers after the huge impact of the Napoleonic wars, and was based on international conferences for important issues involving actions and decisions beyond national borders. The Concert of Europe reinforced international diplomacy and governments became accustomed to high-level meetings and negotiations to avoid military conflicts. It paved the way to the major international conferences that took place during the second half of the century, as mentioned in a Chapter 2.[4]

During the process of reorganising the international system, two fundamental conferences were held in The Hague (1899 and 1907). They marked a new step to reinforce international law for the peaceful settlement of disputes. Moreover, the technical and scientific developments that took place during the nineteenth century, pushed the states towards increased cooperation on medical policies and scientific issues, contributed to the establishment of standards, and the settling of common rules. In transport and communications, regulations for public health policies and international trade were supervised. The Central Commission for the Navigation on the Rhine (1815) and the Danube Commission (1856) began regulating river navigation and are often considered the first international organisations, followed by the International Telegraph Union (1865), the International Bureau of Weights and Measures (1875), and the Universal Postal Union (1878). All of these organisations illustrate the initial development of international technical cooperation.

Pacifist activism also became an increasingly international movement with the organisation of conferences that periodically brought together participants from different nationalities. Contacts sometimes led to the creation of permanent organisations, such as the Inter-Parliamentary Union (1889), to promote diplomacy between national parliaments. The International Peace Bureau (1891) was also established to coordinate the activities of national peace groups. International diplomacy and the pacifist movement had a direct influence on the creation of the League of Nations Society (Great Britain, 1915) and this was the first organisation to promote the idea of international action and diplomatic negotiation to resolve differences inside the limits of peaceful agreements. Similarly, in France, Léon Bourgeois published an essay entitled *Pour la Société des Nations* (1909)[5] and founded the *Association Française pour la Société des Nations* (1918). This international context and the predominant attitude among the big powers had an important influence on Woodrow Wilson, president of the United States of America, and considered as founding father of the League of Nations.

Previous chapters show to what extent the reconstruction of a new international order to challenge conflicts started before the First World War. European initiatives such as those mentioned in France and Great Britain helped convince governments and influence the public opinion. However, the key moment was the speech given by President Wilson before the American Congress in January 1918, in which he stated the 14 points giving political legitimacy to a radical reform of international order. Wilson outlined the necessity of building a peace without victors, rebuilding a new order based on democratic principles, respect for national self-determination, and the abolishment of secret diplomacy. This required the foundation of a 'general association of nations' able to ensure the independence and territorial integrity of states. The negotiations that led to the creation of the League of Nations were conducted at the Peace Conference held in Paris in January 1919. Wilson's viewpoints were opposed by the political interests of the European powers, who were in favour of an international order based on political negotiation and alliance. Nevertheless, the American president finally overcame resistance and imposed his ideas.

The International Labour Organisation (ILO) and the Permanent Court of International Justice were also founded at the Paris Peace Conference in 1919. The Covenant of the League of Nations highlighted its importance in the new international order. From a political perspective, it ensured acceptance from all participating countries at the Peace Conference, but the Covenant became the subject of much political bargaining and the League was assigned responsibilities it was not originally intended to address – such as monitoring treaties on the protection of minority rights and the coordination of the fight against health catastrophes, famine, and medical relief. Moreover, it linked the League to the peace agreements, a decision that was heavily criticised in Germany and Italy (who rejected conditions imposed by the peace treaties). Furthermore, despite Wilson's commitment, the senate in Washington refused to ratify the Treaty of Versailles (March, 1920) and so the American president who led the peace negotiations did so aware of the extent and consequences of the growing isolationist trend at home. Unfortunately, he suffered a stroke after his return to America from Paris and could not defend his viewpoints. The agreement, initially supported by Washington, was finally not signed by the American government. This decision affected the credibility, scope, and effectiveness of the League of Nations from the beginning. Although it was proclaimed to be global, the League was born apart from its principal promoter and a major international power; the United States.

The covenant was the founding treaty of the League, mainly conceived to promote international cooperation in specific technical areas. A series of subsidiary bodies institutionalised cooperation among states and developed international conventions in various fields such as the control of epidemics, public health regulations, the fight against opium and drugs consumption, communications and transit, trafficking in women and children, intellectual cooperation, economy, and humanitarian issues.[6] In certain cases, those bodies provided direct assistance to the states by helping in the fight against epidemics, reorganising healthcare systems, and instructing experts in public health. The distribution of information about social and medical issues played an essential role in the diplomatic action of the League.

International agencies and philanthropic intervention during the first half of the twentieth century contributed to promoting and expanding capitalism, medical technologies, and imperialist strategies, and so also expanded the assumption that political authorities should have a commitment to the improvement of public health, civil rights, welfare, healthcare, and social development.[7] Technical expertise associated with national and international organisations operated to legitimise international intervention and influence national policies, and it was the national authorities who often requested expert advice, or even financial support, to respond to humanitarian tragedies involving epidemics, infections, famine and medical care.

The shift to social medicine involved a growing reliance on national and international experts as independent technical authorities acting on political guidelines.[8] Humanitarian intervention and medical activism became an active movement in Western countries at a time of deep crisis and social conflict.[9] This proved to be a bone of contention in the US during the first decades of the twentieth century.[10] Some organisations such as the League of Red Cross Societies viewed mercy and humanitarian relief as an essential value of medical ethics, above and beyond any assessments of a political character. Yet, several other humanitarian medical associations that emerged during the interwar period believed in actively participating in the struggle between democracy, fascism, and socialism.[11] For instance, medical activism represented by the International Brigades in the Spanish Civil War required political commitment rather than technical neutrality and, to some extent, activists applied the moral imperative of humanitarian relief beyond narrow, real-political interests. The debate mainly revolved around the need to fight for democracy at a time when it was threatened by fascist expansion. In other cases, there was support for the expansion of communism as a global revolution. This wide landscape and the plurality of participants meant that, during the first decades of the twentieth century, social medicine and the international sanitary relief movements were not only matters of imperialist or capitalist expansion.

Recent historiography offers a controversial debate about the aims and impact of the American philanthropic movement, both domestically and internationally. Furthermore, the health politics and social medicine strategies promoted by the Rockefeller Foundation International Health Board/Division and the Health Committee/Health Organisation of the League of Nations, both contributed to the formulation of national health policies and health administration bodies in many countries worldwide, demonstrating a growing engagement of state administrations in the implementation of social medicine strategies.[12]

During the interwar years, experts educated at internationally leading public health institutions and bacteriological research laboratories in various countries, exerted unprecedented technical and ideological influence. International networks increased state involvement in the design and implementation of an expanded *biopolitics*. This was the antecedent leading to the welfare state policies that were developed during the Cold War.

After World War One, many governments organised national public health services as a necessity for the implementation of active health policies, but one of the main grounds for their initial failure was the lack of patterns of organisation and deficient technical expertise. Therefore, diplomatic and financial cooperation with foreign health authorities and policy makers became essential for the successful management and coordination of preventive and sanitary campaigns. Transnational expertise in public health strategies was indeed supported by national authorities, international powers, and health organisations and became a key reference for national health policies.[13] International expertise was not always accepted. When dealing with specific issues, national independence was claimed, and this applies to the publication of national epidemiological records or vaccination campaigns.

Nevertheless, an international consensus regarding the importance of public health experts for efficient state administration was easily generated. As said, previous public health initiatives were independently established by national governments. International campaigns to cope with malaria, hookworm disease, and other health problems, were promoted by the Rockefeller Foundation International Health Board in various countries from the 1920s. The main scope was the creation of technical expertise in statistical evidence – especially in the organisation of national epidemiological services. Laboratory research also served as a basis for vaccination and preventive actions and this was complemented by technical knowledge and practical training in the field. These public health experts became the elite of the national health administrations, and would act as authoritative references for national health services and policies.[14] They formed a network of influential actors.

Some specific events played a prominent role in the shaping of international networks. As we know, a health crisis emerged at the end of World War One. The main risk was represented by epidemic outbreaks – with typhus threatening Eastern European countries weakened by scarcity, migrations, and famine.[15] The Polish government officially applied to the League of Nations in 1919 for the immediate convocation of a Pan-European Conference in Warsaw. It was urgent, to assess the deteriorating situation and prevent the infection spreading westwards by creating a *cordon sanitaire* around the most infected territories on both sides of the borders between Russia and Ukraine and Poland and Rumania. The conference was announced and technical representatives from 20 European governments attended. Despite tensions inside the American political chambers, the United States Public Health Service was also represented. But international relations were seriously damaged by the war and due to the open conflict between Poland and Russia it took four months to bring delegates from both nations together at the conference table. In the opinion of the head of the Health Organisation of the League, Ludwik Rajchman: 'the question now will be to obtain general agreement for the establishment of this *cordon sanitaire*. In our mind, it should consist of concentric lines, epidemic hospitals, quarantine and feeding stations, public baths, and delousing establishments, etc., on both sides of the frontier to a depth of some 150 km'.[16]

Despite a lack of sufficient resources, this strategy was implemented by the governments. The anti-typhus campaign in Poland was considered the first successful effort of international European public health intervention.[17] Rajchman feared that the epidemics may get out of control and so he obtained the collaboration of the Rockefeller Foundation to develop an international perspective regarding the fight against epidemics in such critical moments. The American foundation was also engaged in the fight against malaria, trachoma, and other diseases. The consolidation of the League of Nations Health Organisation thus accelerated the development of networking in the coordination of transnational health policies. Sanitary diplomacy developed collaboration among nations and services, and homogenised public health policies in accordance with new hegemonic groups of experts. The new landscape increased the Rockefeller Foundation's influence over public health politics and initiatives worldwide.

In the context of intense international diplomacy, public health experts became an essential tool for political and social stabilisation, and for negotiating solutions to the health problems affecting various countries. Expert committees shaped policies based on interchange programmes, participation in technical commissions, research groups, and international conferences. An extensive network of people, diplomatic action, and political interventions on health issues took shape. Emergency situations during and after the war justified political reactions to avoid the foreseeable health catastrophes. Moreover, the expansion of national systems of social and health insurance drew attention to the social and economic burden represented by avoidable diseases and called for national regulations and transnational coordination. Once the League of Nations Health Organisation came to be recognised as an agent for the League's stabilisation policies, it shaped an international timeline to eliminate diseases considered to be avoidable or preventable.[18] A report published after one decade of public health activity stated that:

> At any time, governments could request the League of Nations Health Organisation to place experts at their disposal in order to carry out specific tasks, produce technical reports, inform or advise on specific issues. Expert opinions were often requested for specific campaigns against malaria, venereal diseases, dengue fever, and other diseases. Sometimes policy makers requested advice on the organisation of the public health administration in rural districts, primary healthcare centres, or even the entire country. Greece, Bolivia, China, Poland, Spain, among others, requested technical advice at various times and on different issues.[19]

As a result of the Warsaw Conference, conventions on quarantines and sanitary arrangements were approved in 1922 and the implementation of the resolutions was left to the International Epidemic Commission established in June 1920 under the League. This International Epidemic Commission was the first international body endowed with the capacity to make decisions and act in those cases in which two or more nations were affected by a sanitary hazard. The commission had more than an advisory role and was formed as a consequence of the growing awareness of the international dimension of post-war epidemics and the foreseeable demographic catastrophes.[20]

The influential Epidemic Commission included Thorvald Madsen, Director of the *Staten Serum Institut* in Copenhagen, as well as the President of the League of Nations Health Committee; George Buchanan, Senior Medical Officer at the British Ministry of Health and Vice-President of the League's Health Committee; Josephus Jitta, President of the Dutch Hygiene Council; Ricardo Jorge, Director General of the Portuguese Public Health Administration; and Dr Violle, an expert from the Pasteur Institute in Paris. The commission prepared a new International Sanitary Convention that would study existing quarantine arrangements and draft new international agreements. The international context had changed considerably from the nineteenth century – when the existing sanitary agreements had been drafted. Diplomacy was present as well, but the technical body of experts had gained power and influence. Powerful international elites of experts had expanded and coordinated public health and social medicine strategies.[21]

Public health programmes promoted by the Rockefeller Foundation in various nations were predicated on the creation of both international and national professional elites closely linked to the health administration. These elites would found their expertise on the organisation and management of statistical evidence, research on laboratory technologies applied to public health campaigns, preventive measures, and practical training in the field. They had the profile needed to serve as authoritative references for national policies and state health administrations. An important element in this process was the compilation and diffusion of epidemiological information. The League of Nations enthusiastically supported this initiative, and immediately after its creation started to collect data, prepare epidemiological statistics, and circulate periodic reports.[22] The League set up a Service of Epidemiological Intelligence and Public Health Statistics in 1921 for tracking plagues and infectious diseases. In July 1923, the first *Bulletin Mensuel de Renseignements Épidémiologiques* was published, and the service continued producing up-to-date and useful information for national health administrators. From the end of 1923 the monthly reports, appropriately verified and supplemented, were collected and published in an annual report, initially published as *Rapport Épidémiologique Annuel*.[23] The growing importance of the information spread by this international epidemiological service led in 1922 to a request by the Japanese representative that the League also survey the epidemiological situation in the Far East (as it was doing in Eastern Europe).[24] Monitoring the situation in the Far East involved the foundation of a coordinating office similar to the one operating in Geneva. An initial epidemiological survey on the Far East was published in 1922–1923, and later an Office for Epidemiological Information for Asia operated in Singapore from 1925 until the dissolution of the League in 1946.

Statistical information about the impact of diseases and the sanitary situation in any country required technical standardisation to make it comparable. The topic needed to be focused, once more, from a coordinated transnational perspective. Between 1923 and 1925 several expert committee meetings, involving the heads of European epidemiological services, took place with the aim of planning a comprehensive global health report.[25] Common rules for the recording of the registers of diagnosis and causes of death were essential. Therefore the League, together with the International Institute of Statistics, produced in 1929 an important update of the *International List of Causes of Death*, an essential tool for the homologation of epidemiological information, which continues to be revised and used.[26] Initiatives on epidemiological records made governments and national authorities aware of the importance of epidemiology for public health policies.

An International Health Yearbook, or *Annuaire Sanitaire International*, was published in French and English in 1925 with information from 22 countries.[27] It was an initial effort. National authorities sent updated reports on demographic and epidemiologic records, the implementation of sanitary reforms in each country, preferential public health policies, and detailed information about social diseases.[28] Most of those reports seem to be clearly deficient, but, once more, the initiative heightened the perception among governments and health authorities that disease and health conditions should be registered and measured as a starting point for social health policies. The International Health Yearbook was published for five years (1925–1930). It contained valuable information on the international health situation. In 1929, 37 countries contributed information to the publication.[29] However, deficiencies in the planning and technical coordination of the information requested, and also in methodological and linguistic standardization, made the results heterogeneous and so limited their usefulness. The world economic situation deteriorated sharply after 1929 and Rockefeller funding was cut, and so the 1930 volume was the last published.

The *International Health Yearbook* summarised and compiled national reports without further comparative evaluation or transnational analysis. Reports offered demographic and epidemiologic data and information about institutions, facilities, sanitary staff, healthcare, medical insurance, and other topics regarding public health in each country. One of its main contributions was the establishment of a framework of circulating international information that was available to national and international experts. This international epidemiological experience was an excellent instrument to detect problems, discuss solutions, and agree health policies. Measuring the health situation in any nation reinforced the necessity for national offices managed by epidemiologists with technical expertise. Dispensaries for the prevention and treatment of tuberculosis and venereal diseases, campaigns against malaria and other infectious diseases, surveys on the health status of the population, as well as nutritional deficiencies in rural areas were mainly identified according to the establishment of epidemiological information.

Creating expert knowledge

Social medicine increasingly became a transnational issue and a cornerstone for the training of public health experts. These experts were to become the technical actors for a national and international implementation of health policies. Several lines of action took place. One was to collect and publish information on national services and programmes (including how healthcare services were organised and how they operated in several European countries), workplace sanitary regulations, the identification of health problems in each region, and the private and public institutions involved in healthcare and social medicine.[30] A second line of action was to promote exchanges and interactions between countries by funding visits by public health experts to study and discuss specific diseases, learn new technologies, learn how healthcare systems were organised, as well as to learn about the most important facilities and campaigns implemented in several countries.[31] The programme of interchange of public health experts was one of the most important activities implemented by the collaborative programme signed by the Rockefeller Foundation and the League of Nations – and revealed a clear hierarchy where British, American, and French institutions occupied a dominant role.[32]

The first experimental interchange of experts took place in Belgium and Italy between October and December 1922, following grants from the International Health Board of the Rockefeller Foundation. From 1923, various activities involved public health officers, others were conceived for specific issues such as health policies and sanitary campaigns to fight tuberculosis, promote infant hygiene, introduce school hygiene and school medical inspection, organise local and national health administration units, such as port stations, and organise demographic and epidemiologic statistical services in all nations. Despite the permanent financial problems suffered by the League of Nations, the interchanges followed year after year and were presented as one of the most successful initiatives of the League's Health Organisation from the mid-1920s until the 1930s. A well-structured network of leadership in public health interchanges had given visibility and influence to the League and the Rockefeller Foundation. The Conference of Malariologists (1924) gathered the most important international researchers on malaria and experts in preventive and therapeutic policies and so represented a worldwide approach to the problem.

Another interchange of experts was arranged from March until May 1925, involving major cities in the United States. The working topics included rural health, municipal sanitation, malaria research, industrial plants, public health instruction, welfare institutions, health administration, the fight against typhoid fever and hookworm disease control, visits to the Johns Hopkins School of Public Health, sanitation facilities, children's health – including children's bureaus and hospitals – veterinary inspection, management of slaughterhouses, quarantine stations, immigrant medical examinations, and health facilities. The list of issues included in what could be considered social medicine was exhaustive. A long tour was focused on involving Latin American leaders in public health intervention, the main purpose being the implementation of sanitation programmes in those nations. The Johns Hopkins School of Public Health – funded by the Rockefeller Foundation – served as a training institution for foreign fellows of the American foundation.

Various types of collective interchanges were organised by the League – with the most common being that of health officers. The meetings were partially financed by the national governments and the Rockefeller-League. Some focussed on particular issues, and gathered specialists such as health officers from maritime stations in the Mediterranean and Baltic, tuberculosis officers, sanitary engineers, medical school inspectors, and malaria experts. The malaria courses were an offshoot of this system of interchanges. Trained experts were needed in many countries and the League supported malaria courses at national health institutes in Hamburg, London, and Paris, complemented with practical field training in countries affected by malaria: such as Italy, Spain, and Yugoslavia.

The programme for 1926 included interchanges in Great Britain and Denmark.[33] The interchanges in Great Britain were restricted to municipal health officers. The programme consisted of visits made to London institutions and to several counties. Sanitary engineering was a central issue for social policies. An interchange of engineers was planned in London at the same time with the assistance of members of the Royal Sanitary Institute. It is worthwhile noting the importance of interdisciplinary collaboration between a series of professionals taking part in this growing *biopolitical* movement and who were active in social medicine and public health intervention: architects, engineers, doctors, teachers, administration managers, nurses, school inspectors, and veterinaries.

The principal ideologist and defender of this programme of public health expertise interchange was Ludwik Rajchman. He insisted that the League and Rockefeller authorities give priority to shaping transnational expertise, and establish strong networks in social medicine. The interchange in July 1926 was restricted to about ten participants from three or four neighbouring countries. The participants were general health officers with specialist interests, and specialist subjects in which two or three of the countries were affected. Therefore, the issues were locally analysed, although the whole group worked together for the consideration of problems that were important to all the nations.[34]

Between 1922 and 1927 collective interchanges were held in a wide series of territories in all continents: Algeria, Austria, Belgium, Canada, Cuba, Czechoslovakia, Dahomey, Danzig, Denmark, Egypt, France, Gambia, Germany, Gold Coast, Great Britain, Greece, French Guinea, Portuguese Guinea, Hungary, Italy, Ivory Coast, Japan, Korea, Latvia, Manchuria, Netherlands, Nigeria, Norway, Palestine, Poland, Senegal, Kingdom of the Serbs, Croats and Slovenes, Sierra Leone, Spain, Sudan, Sweden, Switzerland, Syria, Togoland and the United States of America.[35] The participants in the activities were drawn from 52 countries, 13 colonies and protectorates, and two mandate territories. In addition, 57 medical officers from 30 countries were selected to study certain pressing problems on individual bases. Experts from Asia studied the method of preparing and administering anti-cholera vaccines in the countries and laboratories where these methods were developed. In addition, Japanese experts in nutrition were given the opportunity to study advances in the science of nutrition as developed in Western laboratories, and specialists in branches of public health administration examined new methods from other countries. The internationalisation programme for public health policies reached worldwide.[36]

According to the reports prepared by the League, the transnational work achieved in public health by 1930 was impressive: 'six hundred officials belonging to state members of the League, and also to non-member states – such as the United States of America, Mexico, and the USSR – had participated in interchanges of health personnel. Nearly all countries in Europe, as well as Latin America, the United States, Canada, West Africa, India, and Japan, have been visited and have sent their officials on study tours'.[37] International diplomacy was established and technical expert networks were in action.

The interchange programme was maintained during the whole period of collaboration between the Rockefeller Foundation and the League. It succeeded in creating a wide network of exchanges and synergic interactions. Between 1923 and 1931 the Health Organisation implemented 35 interchanges for collective study, involving 31 countries with the participation of 587 health officers from 61 countries.[38] The figures reveal the huge dimension of this ambitious initiative and show the political importance of health policies in time of crisis.

When the interchange programme was again evaluated in 1931, one of the most appreciated achievements was having brought the health services of different countries into closer relationship with each other, and so facilitating comparative studies about health organisation and legislation. In sum, the interchange programme of experts contributed a silent transnational expansion of ideas, technologies, problem selections, and political actions. The organisation of every interchange included the preparation of a handbook of the medical and health services of the visited country and detailed reports (which the participants were requested to prepare). The circulated information shaped ideas and attitudes in a context of cooperation.[39] Most national administrations benefited from this experience.

Public health experts as transnational actors

The various public health programmes supported and funded by the International Health Board/Division of the Rockefeller Foundation were intended to create both international and national professional public health experts who could exercise a transnational influence. With close collaboration with the former, the League of Nations amplified its transnational influence. Being an international agency endowed with national representation, the potentially dominating role and interests of the big powers were diluted. These elites of transnational health experts legitimated their expertise on well-defined postgraduate courses based on statistical evidence, experimental, and technical knowledge – as well as practical field training. Schools of public health for sanitary staff were established to serve as authoritative references for state policies and national health services. Trained diplomats were instructed in accordance to international patterns and had a detailed knowledge of public health organisations and strategies implemented in different countries.

National governments maintained full independence with regard to internal policies. However, political decisions depended to a large degree on technical advisory bodies occupied by health officers, who shared a style of scientific thinking, a common technical culture, and similar training to other experts from other nations. They shared information and expertise, discussed new initiatives, and generated information about health conditions and social problems related to disease. An important element in this process – the compiling and diffusion of epidemiological information – was strongly stimulated by the international institutions involved: including the League of Nations, Rockefeller Foundation, *Office Internationale d'Hygiène Publique,* the International Labour Office, and Red Cross societies.

The League of Nations Health Organisation started to collect data and circulate periodic reports that included data from most nations worldwide. A milestone in the internationalisation of public health policies took place in 1921, when the organisation's Health Committee set up a Service of Epidemiological Intelligence and Public Health Statistics in Geneva for tracking plagues and recording infectious diseases subject to compulsory notification. It was conceived as a sort of global warning system and a service capable of mapping the distribution of social diseases worldwide. In the context of this political and institutional expansion, the expert networks played a prominent role of intermediation between politicians, international agencies, transnational research groups, and the big powers.

Notes

1 Boyce, R. *The Great Interwar Crisis and the Collapse of Globalisation*, Hampshire: Palgrave MacMillan, 2012.
2 Swaan, A. de *In Care of the State: Health Care, Education and Welfare in Europe and the USA in the Modern Era*, Oxford: Polity Press, 1988; Flora, P. (ed.) *State formation, nation-building and mass politics in Europe. The theory of Stein Rokkan*, Oxford: Oxford University Press, 1996; Andresen, A.; Hubbard, W.; Ryymin, T. (eds) *International and Local Approaches to Health and Health Care*, Oslo: Novus Press, 2010; Borowy, I; Gruner, W.D. (eds) *Facing Illness in Troubled Times. Health in Europe in the Interwar Years 1918–1939*, Frankfurt am Main: PIE Peter Lang, 2005.
3 Swaan, *In Care of the State* (1988), pp. 10–15; Rabier, Ch. (ed.) *Fields of Expertise: A Comparative History of Expert Procedures in Paris and London, 1600 to Present*, Newcastle: Cambridge Scholars Publishing, 2007; Trentman F.; Just F. (eds) *Food and Conflict in Europe in the Age of the Two World Wars*, New York: Palgrave, 2006.
4 Barona, *The Rockefeller Foundation* (2015).
5 Bourgeois, L. *Pour la Société des Nations*, Paris: E. Fasquelle, 1909.
6 Rodríguez-García, M.; Rodogno, D.; Kozma, L. (eds) *The League of Nations' Work on Social Issues*, Geneva: United Nations, 2016.
7 Rosenberg, E.S. *Spreading the American Dream: American Economic and Cultural Expansion, 1890–1945*, New York: Hill & Wang, 1982; Petersen, K.; Stewart, J.; Sørensen, M.K. (eds) *American Foundations and the European Welfare States*, Odense: University of Odense, 2013.
8 Barona Vilar, J.L. 'Public Health Experts and Scientific Authority'. In Andresen, A.; Hubbard, W.; Ryymin, T. (eds) *International and Local Approaches to Health and Health Care*, Oslo: Novus Press, 2010, pp. 31–48; Rabier (ed.), *Fields of Expertise* (2007), pp. 8–12.
9 Berliner, H.S. *A System of Scientific Medicine: Philanthropic Foundations in the Flexner Era*, New York & London: Tavistock, 1985; Page, B.B.; Valone, D.A. (eds) *Philanthropic Foundations and the Globalization of Scientific Medicine and Public Health*, Lanham: University Press of America, 2007.
10 Landrum, R.B.; Smith, C. *Private Foreign Aid: US Philanthropy for Relief and Development*, Boulder, CO: Westview Press, 1982; Bremner, R.H. *American Philanthropy*, Chicago: University of Chicago Press, 1988; Friedman, L.J.; McGarvie, M.D. (eds) *Charity, Philanthropy, and Civility in American History*, Cambridge: Cambridge University Press, 2003; Tournès, L. 'La philanthropie américaine, la Société des Nations et la coproduction d'un ordre international (1919–1946)', *Relations Internationales*, 151, 2012, pp. 25–36.
11 Wetherby, A. *The Medical Activists: Humanitarians, Activists, and American Medical Relief to Spain and China, 1936–1949*, PhD Thesis, University of Oxford, 2014; Birn, A.E.; Brown, Th. (eds) *Comrades in Health: US Health Internationalists, Abroad and at Home*, New Brunswick: Rutgers University Press, 2013.
12 Löwy, I.; Zylberman, P. 'Introduction. Medicine as a Social Instrument: Rockefeller Foundation, 1913–45', *Studies in the History and Philosophy of Biology and Biomedical Sciences*, 31 (3), 2000, pp. 365–379; Farley, J. *To Cast Out Disease. A History of the International Health Division of the Rockefeller Foundation (1913–1951)*, Oxford: Oxford University Press, 2004.

13 Barona, *The Rockefeller Foundation* (2015), pp. 16–21.
14 Rajchman, L.W. *The League of Nations Health Organisation: What it is and how it works?* Terrytown, New York: RAC, 18 November 1921, RG 1.1, Series 100, Box 20, Folder 165.
15 Rajchman, L.W. 'Report on the Epidemic Situation in Eastern Europe', RAC, RG 1.1, Series 100, Box 20, Folder 165, 18 February 1922.
16 Rajchman, 'Report on the Epidemic Situation (1922),' p. 2.
17 Barona, *The Rockefeller Foundation*, 2015, chapter 2.
18 *Ten Years of World Co-operation* . . . Secretariat of the League of Nations in Geneva, London: Hazell, Watson & Viney, 1930.
19 Barona Vilar, J.L.; Bernabeu-Mestre, J. *La Salud y el Estado. El movimiento sanitario internacional y la administración española (1851–1945)*, Valencia: Publicaciones de la Universidad de Valencia, 2008.
20 Barona, *The Rockefeller Foundation* (2015), pp. 81–90.
21 Rose, W. 'Epidemic control in Europe, and the League.' *American Review of Reviews*, 46, 1922, p. 2; Zinsser, H. 'Report on Journey to Russia as Epidemic Commissioner of Hygienic Section, League of Nations, from June 11 to July 20, 1923,' Terrytown, New York: RAC, RG 1.1, Series 100, Box 22, Folder 183.
22 Barona, J.L. *The Rockefeller Foundation*, 2015, pp. 87–89.
23 *Rapport Épidémiologique Annuel*, Genève: Société des Nations, 1923, pp. 8–9.
24 Barona, J.L. *The Rockefeller Foundation*, 2015, p. 90.
25 'Report of the Health Committee to the Permanent Committee . . .', Geneva: LONA, A.22.1924.III.
26 Borowy, I. 'World Health in a Book – The International Health Yearbooks.' In I. Borowy and W.D. Gruner (eds) *Facing Illness in Troubled Times. Health in Europe in the Interwar Years 1918–1939*, Frankfurt am Main: PIE Peter Lang, 2005, pp. 85–12.
27 The countries participating were: Germany, Austria, Belgium, Bulgaria, Canada, Czechoslovakia, Spain, Estonia, Finland, France, Greece, Hungary, Lithuania, the Netherlands, Norway, Poland, Kingdom of the Serbs, Croats and Slovenes, Romania, Sweden, USA and the USSR.
28 'Instruction to all the States, 14.01.1925 by Rajchman,' LoN Archives, 12B/42592/41461/ Box R953/1919–1927.
29 Borowy, I., *Coming to Terms with World Health. The League of Nations Health Organisation 1921–1946*, Frankfurt am Main, Peter Lange, 2009, p. 91.
30 Rajchman, L.W. 'Instruction to all the States, 14.01.1925 by Rajchman.' Geneva: LONA, 12B/42592/41461/Box R953/1919–1927. See also 'Bibliography of the technical work of the Health Organisation of the League of Nations, 1920–1945', *Quarterly Bulletin of the Health Organisation of the League of Nations*, 15, 1945, pp. 1–235.
31 Barona, J.L. *The Rockefeller Foundation*, 2015, chapter 2.
32 Ibidem.
33 'Letter from S. Gunn to F.F. Russell,' Terrytown, New York: RAC, RG 1.1, series 100, box 20, folder 169, 23 October, 1925; Barona Vilar, J.L. *Food Inspection in Denmark. Reports on meat and milk presented to the League of Nations on the occasion of the visit of European Health Officers in 1924*, Estrup: Danish Agricultural Museum, 2015.
34 Ibidem.
35 Rajchman, L.W. *Review of the Experience*, 1927, p. 7.
36 Aldous, Ch.; Suzuki, A. *Reforming Public Health in Occupied Japan, 1945–52. Alien prescriptions?* London and New York: Routledge, 2012.
37 *Ten Years of World Co-operation* . . . (1930), p. 243.
38 Ibidem, p. 3.
39 Ibidem, p. 5.

4 The relevance of international organisations

Transnational actors guiding health research and health policies: the historical context of national health institutes

International health cooperation started during the nineteenth century as a diplomatic initiative to control the spread of communicable diseases and avoid damaging the interests of the great European powers.[1] The first agreements on health matters among national authorities of different countries were also prompted by the need for measures to protect trade and, at the same time, prevent the spread of disease, particularly cholera, plague, and yellow fever.[2] From the central decades of the nineteenth century, public health regulations derived from political decisions occupied an important place in the international agenda.[3] As discussed in previous chapters, the foundation of several international sanitary networks influenced national and local policies. Transnational bodies and organisations, formal or informal, influenced the lines of development in the production of medical knowledge, strengthened several aspects of clinical practice, and shaped national public health policies and sanitary campaigns. Preventive medicine efforts and most national initiatives for healthcare organisations in urban and rural districts were closely linked with technical reports and advice given by these transnational experts.[4]

International diplomacy around preventive medicine and the fight against epidemics and infections played a prominent role in this process of international collaboration and negotiation. The increasingly widespread political concern about the negative effects of poor health on social stability and national economies also influenced in the foundation of several international scientific organisations in the field of hygiene, health policies, tuberculosis, venereal diseases, children's and mothers' health, feeding and nutrition. The international crisis meant that organisations and initiatives were endowed with growing importance in various domains. The constitutional recognition of health as a civil right in most European nations demanded political commitment and action. Therefore, the emergence of international networks of expertise contributed new forms of political and scientific legitimacy. The interactions between national authorities and international experts opened forms of negotiation around key issues (such as biological and therapeutic standards). These negotiations gave impetus for the creation of national laboratories, institutes, schools of public health, sanitary campaigns, the establishment of expert committees, and the organisation of international conferences. Technical reports and sanitary interventions in national and transnational territories became more common. Most practical uses of science within public policies were linked to the growing prestige of expert opinions from advisory bodies for political authorities and practical decision making.[5]

During the second half of the nineteenth century, the main sites of experimental medicine and laboratory research were research institutes, usually attached to universities, as well as the national agencies that were founded in most European countries. The Pasteur Institute in Paris, the Institute of Hygiene and Tropical Medicine in London, the Robert Koch Institute in Berlin, and the State Institute of Serum in Copenhagen, were among the most representative of these state research institutions for research in public health. In the United States, public health schools and research centres were mostly university institutions. However, in Europe, national research institutions were a mirror for state-national science and medicine. They aimed to institutionalise health policies and experimental research programmes within the framework of the state administration, and were focused on the solution of the most important health problems. These centres had the authority to advise and design preventive medicine. They developed and controlled research programmes on vaccines, sera, immunology technics, and additionally monitored the quality of pharmaceuticals. Over time, they became a venue for scientists from around the world, particularly in Europe. Young scientists began their experimental research in fields such as physiology, serology, bacteriology, or pharmacology following research programmes within transnational networks often linked to those institutions.[6]

After World War One, the process of internationalisation of medical science and the increasing political and commercial importance of agreements on public health were strongly influenced by the International Health Board/Division of the Rockefeller Foundation. The agency signed agreements with many national authorities participating in public health campaigns, financed national and local dispensaries and healthcare centres, and funded research institutions and programmes in experimental medicine. In addition to this work with the state administration, the Rockefeller Foundation designed an efficient policy aiming at creating an extensive network of well-connected public health experts in accordance with its predominantly technical and professionalising model.[7]

The second key actor was the Health Organisation of the League of Nations, which prompted an ambitious international health programme by creating expert commissions, promoting international conferences, exchanging programmes and experiences, encouraging research in certain fields, and funding health campaigns.[8] Both institutions gave a strong impulse to epidemiological research and organised expert knowledge on nutrition, famine, drug consumption, rural hygiene, maternal and child health, standardisation of biological and pharmaceuticals products, and intervened in the fight against infectious diseases such as malaria, tuberculosis, and venereal diseases. The strategy of improving the health standards of the European population was an essential element of international stabilisation policies in a time of huge social tensions and deep international conflicts.[9]

National health institutes or state institutes of hygiene were the names adopted by national institutions established in most Western countries around the turn of the twentieth century. Some were mainly dedicated to emergent experimental serology and bacteriology and researched sera and vaccines to fight infectious diseases. Nevertheless, they were not the only institutions devoted to medical research. Their most relevant attribute – despite some exceptions – was their creation as public institutions to improve the health of the nation. The social organisation of scientific and medical research had obviously national peculiarities and differing traditions. The German university model, for instance, was precisely founded on university research institutes and laboratories, but this was not the case in Spain, France, or the United States.

However, once the state and the public administration assumed the responsibility to improve the health of the nation, this commitment required institutionalisation. National institutes researched public health problems and set regulatory norms for vaccines, prioritising the fight against the most urgent health problems, obtaining and analysing epidemiological records, and regulating measures to avoid intrusion, quackery, and bad healthcare practice. In Europe, national institutes of hygiene shared common goals and similar patterns. They were all active agents in a new age in which the health of the population, the state, and experimental science articulated the ties that bound together scientific concepts, medical practice, and social and political intervention. National institutes were the key instruments for social medicine and *biopolitics*. Their legitimacy was mainly based on the application of laboratory technologies to challenge social problems, which were previously dimensioned by epidemiological surveys. Clinical checking, medical research, and social information were the elements to formulate appropriate political responses. Experimental laboratory techniques played an essential role as a powerful instrument for transforming, identifying, and conceptualising disease, as well as exploring the body, identifying and defining risks, and isolating hazards.[10]

The main objective of these national institutes was coordinating the implementation of social hygiene as an essential part of state policies. In practical terms, this meant challenging social problems derived from poverty, marginality, hunger, and identifying the social and biological factors involved to find experimental and social solutions. It implied, as a first step, mapping the distribution of disease, discovering the main health problems affecting the community, then promoting sanitary campaigns and other measures of treatment and prevention. A series of new investigative methods were developed that complemented laboratory techniques in screening living conditions: vital statistics; social and anthropological surveys on life habits; diet; and epidemiological records. All of these methods contributed new and well-measured information on the social dimension of disease and affected populations. Laboratory analysis identified infectious diseases, nutrition deficiencies, levels of health, and physical development. Other technologies such as sera, vaccines, vitamins, and drugs also played a preventive role. Social research and laboratory medicine were the fundamental elements of the state commitment to public health during the first decades of the twentieth century.

A common pattern of action was established in most European countries to deal with infectious diseases, whose control and eradication was at the core of the emergence of public health as a central feature of modern social politics.[11] Smallpox was the focus in most countries of the first national campaigns of preventive medicine, as happened in the case of Spain and leading in 1871 to the establishment of the *Instituto Nacional de la Vacuna* [National Vaccine Institute], whose main task was to organise and control anti-smallpox vaccination programmes along the lines of similar institutions in France, Germany, and other European countries. It was succeeded in 1894 by the *Instituto Nacional de Bacteriología y de Higiene*, which became the central national health institution covering areas of epidemiology, bacteriology, serum-therapy, vaccination, parasitology, disinfection and veterinary medicine. In 1910 its name was changed to *Instituto Nacional de Higiene Alfonso XIII*.[12] This is a clear example of how between 1871 and 1910 an institution progressively expanded, adapted to state policies, and used the tools developed by experimental research for social hygiene.

The institutional significance of these national institutes is documented by the range of the activities they undertook: registration of anthropometric and racial records in the metropolis and colonial territories; surveying the state of health and welfare of the population; researching the main social diseases (smallpox, leprosy, malaria, tuberculosis, venereal diseases, and sleeping sickness); launching preventive initiatives and campaigns; and the mapping of disease territories. These institutes were advisory bodies and research units at the service of governmental policies. Similar functions were carried out by comparable national health institutes in most Western countries. Was this a simple coincidence or was it a consequence of emulation? Or perhaps a consequence of social reformism implemented by liberal states? The following pages explore how knowledge and technologies produced by experimental medicine were applied to produce scientific knowledge and inspire political practice; and the role played by scientific activities in shaping individual and national identities.[13]

Legitimising arguments: moral values, health, and economy

National health institutions were instruments of the state for implementing new health policies inspired by experimental medicine and social research. They emerged as necessary instruments for state administrations, developing experimental techniques and applying them to achieve a fundamental goal: overcoming poverty and improving living conditions, and thereby relieving suffering and sickness. The link between poverty, degeneration, and infectious disease had been increasingly argued since the Enlightenment. Social and political stability was an important objective. In its report proposing to parliament the establishment of the *Instituto Nacional de Higiene*, the Spanish government cited humanitarian and patriotic reasons as the central justification:

There is an urgent need to study infectious-contagious endemic diseases, currently unattended in Spain, despite thousands of deaths every year; study the serious problems of infection in general, as thousands of laboratories in advanced countries passionately do; study the world of bacteriology and gain knowledge on the most fundamental matters of organic life; instruct and teach disinfection staff to handle with efficiency the national and international requirements in public health; develop lymph vaccine in the proportion required by vaccination demands, which is becoming compulsory, liberate humanity from smallpox, causing many thousands of victims every year in Spain, and safely establish the production of healing and preventive sera against rabies, diphtheria, anthrax, etc. These are very transcendental needs for public health which should be addressed with the proportionate resources obtained from popular subscription when the limited funds contributed by the state are insufficient, since the institute is of general interest and for the benefit of everybody.[14]

Appeals were made to charitable and philanthropic associations to contribute financial and human support to the foundation of a national institute, since bacteriological science enabled medical laboratories to produce sera and vaccines to fight infectious diseases, such as diphtheria, rabies, tetanus, parasitic diseases, puerperal fever, tuberculosis and cholera. Moreover, national medical laboratories not only represented modernity and progress in social imaginary, they were also shown as an important source of state revenue. These economic arguments were raised during the political debates in parliament. Spain paid large sums to buy products from the *Institute Pasteur*, which had demonstrated the benefits of medical-technical laboratories for cattle farming, biotechnologies, ferments, manures, and pest control, as well as making huge contributions to human health. Municipal, provincial, and national medical inspectors – an administrative body of civil servants with expertise in public health issues – managed those institutes. Spanish authorities usually mentioned Imperial Germany's network of laboratories as the model to follow, including the Institute for Tropical Hygiene in Hamburg.[15]

But the development of a bureaucratic network of public health experts required instruction, expertise, and the capacity to manage the functions demanded. Most advanced countries in serological and bacteriological research had, by the end of the nineteenth century, their own programmes, institutions, and groups. Other countries tended to imitate the model. In addition to the state administrations, various international bodies contributed to the foundation of national health institutions in the early twentieth century: including the *Office International d'Hygiène; Publique*, the Rockefeller Foundation; the International Labour Office; and the League of Nations.

Awareness of the economic and social dimension of public health problems prompted the creation, within the Rockefeller Foundation, of an International Health Board to conduct an epidemiological survey and develop a plan of intervention to solve the high incidence of hookworm affecting miners in some American states. The initial project included an extended medical examination, a therapeutic campaign, and a programme of prevention to combat the principal form of spreading the disease: soil contamination by excretes of miners affected by the disease.[16] Five years later, in 1914, 250,000 family houses and more than half a million people in 653 counties had been checked – and nearly 450,000 patients had been treated. This was probably the largest medical screening ever implemented to cope with an occupational disease and it constitutes an excellent example of social medicine and *biopolitics*.

Given the high level of success achieved with this initiative, John D. Rockefeller decided, in May 1913, to create the Rockefeller Foundation with an initial endowment of 100 million dollars. A month later a specialist agency devoted to international public health was established: *International Health Board* [IHB] 'for the purpose of extending the inhabitants of other countries the fight against hookworm disease and ensure that the treatment and healing is accompanied by the founding of agencies to promote public health and the dissemination of knowledge related to scientific medicine'. That was the first and main line of international health intervention pursued by the Rockefeller Foundation for the next ten years, together with other campaigns against malaria and yellow fever.

But the Rockefeller Foundation management became aware of the ephemeral nature of health interventions promoted by private agents when the state was not actively involved. The objective of achieving a worldwide network of public health policies based on institutions and strategies of intervention required the involvement of the nation states, as well as the authority and legitimacy of transnational powers. This gives exceptional importance to the collaboration established between the Rockefeller Foundation and the newly created Health Organisation of the League of Nations.[17] Hence, the International Health Board focused primarily on spreading awareness among political authorities and encouraging public support for national health authorities for teaching experts and establishing well-equipped institutions with experimental facilities. At the same time, the Rockefeller Foundation funded public health departments at American universities to instruct health officers in managing public health strategies. In addition, postgraduate schools of hygiene were declared to be key agencies for conducting health policies in all countries. Its influence over experts and national institutions would make the Rockefeller Foundation a powerful organisation, absolutely hegemonic in transnational public health. Its flagship institution was the Johns Hopkins School of Hygiene in Baltimore.

In accordance with this guidance, action lines were given for the expansion of health policies, negotiation with governments for the establishment of schools of public health, and implementation of campaigns against previously defined social diseases. Obviously, the success of the entire model had a cornerstone: the training of a wide network of public health specialists who were capable of coping with practical measures, researching public health issues, and serving as technical authorities to the liberal state.

The Health Organisation of the League of Nations and the Rockefeller Foundation signed in 1923 an agreement for cooperation in public health, according to which a series of programmes for international health prompted by the League were funded by the American foundation. These included an interchange programme for public health experts, and meetings of directors of national schools of hygiene. Funding from the RF enabled the expansion of new institutions in Madrid, Zagreb, Budapest, Prague, Bucharest, and Warsaw. The whole international strategy was implemented in close negotiation with national governments.

The international programme of exchange for public health experts contributed technical expertise, knowledge about developments in the most advanced countries, new initiatives, and common training and advice for state administrators. These newly trained national elites were then called on to guide national schools and institutes of hygiene, and so constituted a hegemonic network capable of governing state policies and establishing transnational patterns. The power and capacity of influence achieved by the Rockefeller in this domain was so vast and transnational that it controlled global health policies (based on technical parameters) worldwide and left the state governments in a subsidiary role. The leaders of the RF and the League of Nations both agreed that the establishment of national health administrations was essential to cope with social diseases. In January 1923, the Health Committee of the League of Nations resolved to gather the necessary information to make a report on the circumstances of specialised studies in public health and preventive medicine in European, American, and Japanese universities. The proposal reflected confidence that adequate training of public health experts, teaching of hygiene to sanitary staff, and health education for the whole population would improve the health of the population and contribute to social stability by overcoming poverty.[18]

The Health Committee of the League of Nations approved the creation of a specialist standing committee on 20 February 1924, which was named the Commission on Education in Hygiene and Preventive Medicine, and chaired by a specialist representative of the French government, Léon Bernard. The commission consisted of seven members, including the Spanish director of the Madrid institute, Gustavo Pittaluga, who was a member of the Health Committee of the League of Nations, along with other experts and members, to which was added the dean of the Medical School of Shanghai in 1930. From that moment, the RF funded an ambitious programme of international exchanges for public health experts (linked to national governments in Europe, Asia, and America) to discuss and initiate campaigns for health intervention.[19]

Notes

1 Harrison, M. *Contagion. How Commerce has Spread Disease*, Yale: Yale University Press, 2013.
2 Harrison, M. 'Disease, diplomacy and international commerce: the origins of international sanitary regulation in the Nineteenth Century', *Journal of Global History*, 1, 2006, pp. 197–217.

3 Barona Vilar, J.L.; Bernabeu-Mestre, J. *La Salud y el Estado. El movimiento sanitario internacional y la administración española (1851–1945)*, Valencia: Publicaciones de la Universidad de Valencia, 2008.
4 Armitage, D. *Foundations of Modern International Thought*. Cambridge: Cambridge University Press, 2013; Barona Vilar, J.L.; Cherry, S. (eds) *Health and Medicine in Rural Europe (1850–1945)*, Valencia: Publicaciones de la Universidad de Valencia / Seminari d'Estudis sobre la Ciència, 2005.
5 Barona Vilar, J.L. 'Public Health Experts and Scientific Authority'. In Andresen, A.; Hubbard, W.; Ryymin, T. (eds) *International and Local Approaches to Health and Health Care*, Oslo: Novus Press, 2010, pp. 31–48.
6 Barona Vilar, J.L. 'In the Name of Health. The *Instituto Nacional de Higiene Alfonso XIII* and laboratory campaigns in Spanish rural áreas and African colonies, 1910–1924'. In Andresen, A.; Gronlie, T.; Hubbard, W.; Ryymin, T. (eds) *Health Care Systems and Medical Institutions*, Oslo: Novus Press, 2009, pp. 154–169; *Gesundheit schützen, Risiken erforschen. Wer wir sind, Worauf wir zurückblicken, Was wir leisten*, Berlin: Robert Koch-Institut, 2011.
7 Farley, J. *To Cast Out Disease. A History of the International Health Division of the Rockefeller Foundation (1913–1951)*, Oxford: Oxford University Press, 2004.
8 Barona, *The Rockefeller Foundation*, 2015, pp. 28–32.
9 Ibidem.
10 Anderson, W. 'Postcolonial Histories of Medicine.' In F. Huisman and J. Harley (eds) *Locating Medical History: The Stories and their Meanings*, Baltimore: Johns Hopkins University Press, 2004, pp. 285–306; Marks, S. 'What is Colonial about Colonial Medicine? And what has happened to Imperialism and Health?' *Social History of Medicine*, 1, 1997, pp. 205–219; Sutphen, M.P.; Bridie A. (eds) *Medicine and Colonial Identity*, London and New York: Routledge, 2003.
11 Andresen, A.; Barona, J.L.; Cherry, S. (eds), *Making a New Countryside? Health Policies and Practices in European History c. 1860–1950*, Frankfurt am Main: PIE Peter Lang, 2010.
12 Porras Gallo, MI. 'Antecedentes y creación del Instituto de Sueroterapia, Vacunación y Bacteriología Alfonso XIII', *Dynamis*, 18, 1998, pp. 81–106.
13 Medina, R. 'Extracting the Spanish Nation from Equatorial Guinea. Scientific Technologies of National Identity as Colonial Legacies', *Social Studies of Science*, 39, 2009, pp. 81–112.
14 Ministerio de la Gobernación, *Proyecto de un Instituto Nacional de Higiene (Bacteriología. Vacunación. Sueroterapia. Análisis química. Desinfección). Grases, arquitecto*, Madrid: Imprenta Enrique Teodoro y Alonso, 1901.
15 *Proyecto de un Instituto Nacional de Higiene . . .* 1901.
16 *The Rockefeller Foundation: A Digital History. Essays, biographies and thousands of digitalized documents*. Https://rockfound.rockarch.org
17 Barona, *The Rockefeller Foundation* (2015), pp. 18–24.
18 Weindling, P. 'Public health and political stabilisation: The Rockefeller Foundation in Central and Eastern Europe between the two World Wars', *Minerva*, 31, 1993, pp. 253–267.
19 Barona, *The Rockefeller Foundation* (2015), pp. 23–24.

5 Research for the nation
National hygiene institutes

Bacteriology, a cornerstone for colonial medicine

The establishment of national institutes of health showed a common pattern in Western countries around the turn of the twentieth century. The *Institut Pasteur* (1887) in Paris, the Prussian Institute for Infectious Diseases (Robert Koch Institute) (1891) in Berlin, the Lister Institute of Preventive Medicine (1891), the London School of Hygiene and Tropical Medicine (1899) and the Medical Research Council (1913) in London, the Public Health and Marine Hospital Service (1903) in Washington D.C., the *Instituto Nacional de la Vacuna* (1871) and the *Instituto Nacional de Higiene Alfonso XIII* (1900) in Madrid shared aims and political roles. They represented a new age in which, health, the state, and experimental research encompassed the ties that bound together scientific concepts, medical practice, and social and political interventions. The legitimacy of a wide range of national institutions related to health policies was mainly based on the application of clinical and laboratory technologies – blood analysis, body exploration, parasitology, bacteriological and serological technologies – and social surveys based on vital statistics and epidemiology. Under the national institutions were municipal laboratories of bacteriology and chemistry, which took care of infections, water, and food control.

National institutes of hygiene aimed to screen the healthy and the sick, obtaining medical information and formulating appropriate political responses. This chapter discusses how the combination of experimental science and technology, helped by social surveys opened a new stage in social medicine and state *biopolitics*. New expectations emerged regarding the capacity for fighting epidemics and infectious diseases. The new scientific and social worldview of infection, disease, and degeneration was linked to microbes and poverty.[1] Bacteriology appeared as an excellent tool for the screening of colonial territories and rural communities, a space considered to be the origin of most plagues, epidemics, and infectious disease. As agents of social medicine, national institutes of hygiene contributed to shaping the social dimension of health and disease, assessing risk and hazards, and becoming experimental tools for nations and colonial territories. Their foundation was closely linked to the emergence of bacteriological research. The colonies appeared as territories for tropical medicine to prevent epidemics and identify causes.

Moreover, during the interwar years, national research institutions became the main participants, expert agencies for national and international health policies, for the shaping of preventive medicine and social hygiene through the achievements of experimental laboratory techniques based on international expertise. National institutes of hygiene were conceived in accordance with a similar model, although with peculiarities and differences, and they were shaped by a strong diplomatic effort led by international organisations that were almost always funded by the Rockefeller Foundation.

The ideological background to these national institutes of health was *social hygiene*, which meant, broadly speaking, improving the state of health and the health indicators of the population by means of experimental research and active *biopolitics*. This implied, as a first step, mapping the reach and distribution of disease, identifying the principal health problems, and setting *health policies* for sanitary campaigns, as well as other means to cope with infections and preventive medicine. The traditional approach to public health based on water and land sanitation was suddenly insufficient to meet the expectations generated by experimental medicine. New social tools were developed that complemented laboratory techniques in screening conditions: statistics; social and anthropological surveys; and epidemiological records. Experimental research, clinical screening, and health statistics were the main tools for checking the situation facing each society, social group, and disease. This was the background of a new culture, named social hygiene, and the ideological justification of state intervention. Laboratory analysis was to establish patterns of health normality, verify the identification of any infectious disease, nutritional deficiencies, physical development of children and, in some cases, the borders between health and disease. Other technologies such as the production of sera, vaccines, vitamins, and pharmaceuticals also played a preventive role. Public good and health improvement were the main reasons given for action.

Experimental medicine initiated a new age from the perspective of the epistemology of health and disease,[2] and in the political dimension of the fight against diseases. By incorporating laboratory medicine, university research laboratories and national hygiene institutes were endowed with scientific authority and became iconic in the symbolic imagery of modernity and scientific progress. The creation of national health organisations devoted to research, specialist training, and *biopolitics* enabled the state and local administrations to survey and coordinate sanitary campaigns by identifying and defining social diseases. Political initiatives for the control and eradication of infectious disease became a key issue for many Western countries and regions in the transition from the nineteenth to the twentieth century. Modernity was at odds with alcoholism, syphilis, tuberculosis, and high infant mortality rates, and statistics showed the size of the problem and the differences between nations.

A generally common pattern of action was established in most European countries at the core of the emergence of public health as a central feature of state *biopolitics*. Smallpox was, since the eighteenth century, the chief terror susceptible to challenge from national campaigns of vaccination and preventive medicine. The fight against smallpox was a solid argument for the establishment of national institutions of hygiene, whose activities were soon reinforced by new threats: cholera; yellow fever; sleeping sickness; and malaria. These threats were mostly linked to the growing concern of European powers for the colonies and tropical territories.

The establishment of state bureaucracies shaping different forms of health administrations to implement *biopolitics* was closely associated to new developments in the state administration associated with the emergence of health as a political issue. This context led Bruno Latour to explain the transformation of Louis Pasteur as a social and political icon.[3] Latour suggested that it did not matter whether the main characters of the story were scientists, clinicians, microbes, or political administrators.[4] The same could be said in the case of Robert Koch in Germany and Santiago Ramón y Cajal in Spain. Each participant in the network played a specific role depending on power relations. State *biopolitics* in the interwar years represented a plural network of nature, science, and society.

As discussed in a previous chapter, legitimising arguments included moral values, the recognition of health as a civil right, and economic revenue. At a critical time when the nation-state required healthy people to contribute wealth and defend the country in the fight against rival powers, what Latour called *pasteurization* – and we can conceptualise as *public health biopolitics* – became one of the most appropriate solutions.

Indeed, scientific research and the health of the population are linked to the economy, war, and social change[5] – and therefore, health, living conditions, and habits became the most important target for social medicine. In the fight against hunger, mortality, infectious diseases, and the control of epidemics in the colonies, laboratory research was not an autonomous force resulting from the inner dynamic of laboratory work and discoveries. On the contrary, the spread of *biopolitics* and the establishment of health administrations was a result of social crisis and war, where multiple social, economic, political, and cultural forces interconnected. To understand and give a consistent historical explanation to the impulse of experimental public health in the interwar years, we need know nothing more than the power relations between the participants taking part in these complex networks.[6] It is relevant to identify tensions, alliances, and rivalries, and how they struggled and were associated with each other. Everything taking part in the interwar years as a historical context for social hygiene – characters, actions, power relations, programmes, institutions – can better be explained if the main participants are not predetermined. How the network of participants works at a certain historical moment enables us to understand at once the *content* of the experimental grounds of public health and its *context*. Any narrative built through the presentation of the documentary materials does not necessarily follow a lineal diachronic approach, but rather a network of associations that slowly made up the experimental public health universe and its process of institutionalisation.

National institutions were devoted to public health because of active state involvement and intervention in health and disease. During the interwar years, any *biopolitical* issue (hunger, alcoholism, sexuality, prostitution, venereal diseases, tuberculosis, pregnancy, infant mortality, and many others) was typically legitimated by their advocates as necessary instruments to achieve social development, overcome poverty, improve standards of living, and thereby relieve suffering and sickness. The idea of welfare can be glimpsed.

Experimental public health and social medicine flourished in a particular socio-historical context, when liberal socio-political reformism assumed the idea of *regenerating mankind* as a social-political goal. The most powerful agent in the diffusion and translation of public health values was the so-called *hygienism* or *hygienist movement.*[7] If we look at the issue from the perspective of Latour's *actor-network theory*, successful innovation in sera, vaccines, pharmaceuticals, nutrition research, vitamin production and other innovative technologies, was only possible when the diverse and heterogeneous characters – whether they were human or nonhuman – allied with each other to shape a stable, powerful, and actively reinforcing network. When anthrax became pandemic and when cholera epidemics devastated the European population, the most powerful and essential actor in the network was the microbe. Nevertheless, the power relation was reversed as soon as bacteriology, serology, and other instruments of experimental research redefined the social links, achieved greater *biopower*, and then 'became the spokesmen for these new innumerable, invisible, and dangerous agents'[8] by isolating microbes from other actors and making them visible through the microscope using experimental techniques. During the interwar years, it was the health experts associated with diplomats, international agencies, and politicians, who built the new institutions (laboratories, dispensaries, and expert commissions) that transformed scientific experiments into social campaigns and political actions. From the late nineteenth-century, the alliance between statisticians, diplomats, and public health experts using experimental medicine, radically changed the very conception of society, its extent, and capacity for influence.

This network of participants shows how experimental public health achieved sufficient power to rearrange and redefine the actor's positions and the relations and influences in the network. The ideology of the social hygiene programme was the dominance of scientific expertise over nature. Indeed, it implied the supremacy of science and scientific values over society and politics. With the advent of experimental public health, the impact of *biopolitics* left nothing untouched. Latour explains how society could pressure scientists to research the social problem of infectious diseases, but scientists could redefine the whole network through scientific results and innovation, and then science could reverse the direction of pressure and force change in social policies and interventions.[9] Using Latour's words, the presence of the microbe redefined the meaning of individual freedom. Urban reform projects in cities and sanitation in rural districts are good examples, as well as the medicalisation of sexuality and venereal diseases: 'nobody had the right to contaminate others. In order to save everyone's liberty, the contagious patient must be notified by the doctors, isolated, disinfected, and put out of harm's way, like a criminal'.[10] Similar circumstances could be found when dealing with hunger and diet, tuberculosis and alcoholism, and drugs consumption. In many cases, the pressure implied blaming the victim.

Origins and impact of the Pasteur Institute

The Pasteur Institute represents a paradigmatic icon, a model for the new national experimental research institutes. Founded by a decree of 4 June 1887, the Pasteur Institute was inaugurated on 14 November 1888, thanks to the success of an international subscription that enabled Louis Pasteur to institutionalise and extend vaccination against rabies, implement experimental research on a series of infectious diseases, and project scientific knowledge and health technologies as a tool for social development.[11] This was initially a personal initiative of Pasteur himself, supported by international contributions, rather than any academic or state initiative. Indeed, the foundation of the Pasteur Institute in Paris was linked to Pasteur's success in his rabies vaccination experiments and the expectations derived from it. It was on 6 July 1885 that Pasteur administered the anti-rabies vaccine to humans for the first time. He announced to his colleagues from the Académie des Sciences the first successes a year later. More than 350 anti-rabies treatments had been carried out and he called for the creation of a specialised institute to take charge of new research and the production of vaccinations.

Pasteur's desire was to associate research and teaching at a centre for vaccination experimentation and bacteriological research, although the new institution was conceived as a private foundation. He wanted to make it independent of the state administration, but above all, he aimed to ensure that the research institution had a regular income to guarantee its continuity. Given the huge prestige won by Pasteur, the initiative became highly successful and the new foundation raised funds from many sources – French and foreign. The reaction was so enthusiastic that the foundation could buy a plot of land to start the construction of a building for the institute. Two years later, on 4 November 1888, the first building was inaugurated by the French president, a fact that shows the political repercussion of experimental research on public health and the expectations raised by Pasteur's experiments and new bacteriology. The centre housed a vaccination centre, several research laboratories, a library, several lecture rooms, as well as the private apartment of Louis Pasteur. The Institute was divided into five departments: one for rabies research and the other four for basic and applied research.

These initial facilities already highlight some of the chief characteristics of the Pasteur Institute: associating a centre for vaccination with research laboratories and teaching activities. The concept and structure of the new research institute in the late 1880s was substantially different than those built during the interwar years. Serological research and dissemination of new microbiologic techniques was one of the main objectives of the new institute – which served as a French national icon for the international community. Consequently, the Pasteur Institute gained success and prestige, and soon included a hospital, which served as a testing space for the application of new technologies. The Pasteur Institute subsequently made several discoveries and enjoyed the political, financial, and ideological support of the French government and society. It became a place of pilgrimage for bacteriological and serological research by public health experts from around the world. Moreover, it contributed to the French economy by becoming a centre for sera and vaccine production, trade, and exportation.

International impact and profit was one of the principal goals, and the institute exerted great influence on bacteriologists and serologists worldwide. However, the colonies were affected in a more specific way – becoming experimental territories for social medicine research and the implementation of the most recent bacteriological programmes and developments.

Internationalisation was initially attempted in various ways. Firstly, by receiving animals affected by rabies from all over the world and submitting them to experimental vaccination. Many municipal and national laboratories throughout the world learnt and put into practice the new vaccination technologies. From the very beginning, the Pasteur Institute hosted many foreign trainees, mainly led by Pasteur's pupil, Pierre-Paul-Émile Roux. Those public health inspectors went back to their countries, taught the new techniques, and in many cases bought from the Pasteur Institute its products and applied the new technologies in municipal and national health laboratories. This strategy gave the Pasteur Institute great prestige and huge influence. In addition, a strategy of founding a network of sections of the Pasteur Institute overseas widely contributed to its success. Adrien Loir, Pasteur's nephew, founded the first Pasteur Institute in Sydney, Australia, in 1888. In 1891, Albert Calmette founded the Pasteur Institute at Saigon (Vietnam), which was to play a pivotal role in the diffusion of vaccination technologies throughout Indochina: including anti-rabies vaccine, immunisation against smallpox, and anti-venereal serum-therapy.

Three stages could be established in the evolution of the Pasteur Institute from its foundation.[12] The first period extended from its foundation in the 1880s until the First World War (1914–1918). This could be considered as the most successful period of the Institute from a scientific perspective. In the early 1880s, the German doctor Emil Behring and his Japanese assistant Kitasato developed the principle of therapeutic sera. The method was based on the discovery that animals would produce antibodies against most microbial agents when exposed to them, regardless of whether the microbe induced a disease in the animal or not. Such antibodies can be collected from the animals' blood and will kill microbes when injected into a diseased animal or human. Behring and Kitasato discovered that they could exploit this mechanism to produce therapeutic sera against many serious infectious diseases.

During these years, Elie Metchnikoff researched phagocytosis and what today is called cellular immunology. Jules Bordet also developed important research on the role of humoral immunity, and Émile Duclaux – the successor to Louis Pasteur as head of the institute – published work on the functions of enzymes and microbial biological chemistry. The Pasteur Institute contributed fundamental discoveries to the understanding of the biological basis of infection and the biological immunity response in animals and humans. All of these contributions gave the centre international prestige. In addition, the institute also contributed applied methods to public health technologies, which prompted social medicine, and this is more important for the orientation of this book. Experiments by Jules Bordet lead to the development of the so-called Bordet-Wassermann serological test for the detection of syphilis. Émile Duclaux performed research on the composition of milk, and conducted studies on beer and wine with many applications for the development of food industries. This first period was also very rich in medical contributions. The development by Émile Roux and his collaborators in 1894 of anti-diphtheria serum-therapy had a considerable medical and social impact, and gave the Pasteur Institute a leading role for serological laboratories worldwide and for the experimentation of sera and vaccines. When compared with other infections, anti-rabies vaccine in the 1890s was more of a scientific achievement, and a model of successful technology, than a tool demanded by a real health problem. Bacteriology made rabies an imaginary nightmare, but it was not a serious public health problem. Rabies affected only a few individuals, while diphtheria, tuberculosis, influenza, cholera, and syphilis killed thousands.

Numerous Pasteur Institutes were founded in the French colonies in the 20 years following the foundation of the original institute. In addition to those of Sydney and Saigon, already mentioned, branches of the institute were established in Algiers, Tunis, and Tangier in the Maghreb, another in Nha Trang (Indochina), and another in Saint Louis in Senegal. The colonial network of Pasteur Institutes gave a new dimension to its capacities and greatly added to its international public health project. Health technologies not only showed efficiency for curing infections, but also became a source of revenue for the state and private industry.

Colonial territories showed different health problems than those in the European metropolis. Tropical medicine aimed to analyse, screen, and test the influence of environmental and social conditions. The indigenous population served as a test field for new clinical and experimental research and so facilitated new discoveries. Most of the Pasteur Institute contributions benefited from this international expansion through the colonial territories. Alexandre Yersin identified the plague bacillus *(Yersinia Pestis)* in Hong Kong in 1894, and Louis Simond highlighted the role of fleas in the spread of plague in India (1898), Charles Nicolle described the role of lice in the spread of typhus (Tunis, 1909). Albert Calmette developed an anti-venereal serum-therapy in Saigon before moving to Lille after being appointed director of the new Lille Institute Pasteur (founded in 1895). Consequently, the Pasteur Institute became a benchmark for transnational research on serology and bacteriology.

The first stage in the history of the institute ended in 1914 as the war broke up its research programmes. Many researchers were called to the war front and laboratories were mainly reoriented towards the production of vaccines and serums for the troops, or even towards the production of chemical and biological weapons. Furthermore, the global economic crisis following the First World War was to diminish the financial resources of the institute and limit the renewal of researchers, research programmes, and facilities.

Therefore, the impact of the institute declined during the interwar years. Nevertheless, members of the institute participated in numerous international agencies (especially expert commissions of the League of Nations) and the institute took on various new commitments. Researchers from the institute participated in campaigns for the eradication of malaria in Algeria, Italy, Yugoslavia and Spain, as well as in expert commissions for the negotiation of biological standards, epidemics, and other issues. Activities also included active participation in the agreements on regulatory issues for vaccines, vitamins, sera, pharmaceuticals and biological products.

Immunology research had been a flourishing domain during the first years of the institute, especially with the contributions of Elie Metchnikoff. Disagreements and rivalries among his pupils meant that the *Institut Pasteur* did not actively participate in the development of immune-chemistry until after the Second World War. Similarly, Duclaux extended Pasteur's work on fermentation and introduced new *in vitro* techniques. Gabriel Bertrand, Duclaux's successor in the research laboratory and in the chair of biological chemistry, focused his work on the role of complex metal ions in enzymatic catalysis. However, the institute made no contribution to research on metabolic cycles nor to the role of enzymes catalysing biological processes. These were essential elements for the great new paradigms of biochemistry during the first half of the twentieth century.

This second period in the history of the institute also had positive aspects due to a series of brilliant successes in the fight against infectious diseases. Gaston Ramon, a veterinary and photographer introduced several essential practical modifications to the vaccination, highlighting the role of certain compounds named adjuvants in increasing the effectiveness of vaccinations at the Pasteur Institute of Garches (Nanterre, France). The first poly-vaccinations were applied and the technique of formalin inactivation of diphtheria toxin was implemented (which facilitated the production and distribution of anti-diphtheria serum). This new technique enabled the development of the first effective diphtheria vaccine. The institute consolidated its role of exporting sera and vaccines, and also attracted microbiologists and pharmacists from all over the world to learn the technologies of production.

A research line on therapeutic chemistry was also established at the Institute Pasteur from 1911 with the creation of a department of chemistry under Ernest Fourneau. This laboratory made tests on syphilis medications – contributing *stovarsol* – and trials with compounds which were effective against several parasitic diseases prevalent in Africa, particularly against sleeping sickness or trypanosomiasis (*orsanine* and *moranyl*). New compounds of the group of sulfonamides were tested to assess their antibacterial activity, a contribution attributed to Daniel Bovet in 1935. Sulphonamides were later partially eclipsed by the arrival of penicillin, and subsequently, other antibiotics started to be applied to chemotherapy.

Although the second period was not so overwhelmingly successful for the international impact of the Pasteur Institute in Paris, it nevertheless represented a very important moment for the history of the overseas sections of the institute. Let us recall the great campaigns carried out against malaria in French West Africa and in Equatorial Africa colonies by Pasteur researchers (among them Eugene Jamot). Additionally, of great importance was the development of a yellow fever vaccine at the Institute Pasteur in Dakar. The disintegration of the French empire broke up the network of Pasteur institutes and the ties with many were broken. All these factors led to a serious financial crisis, which was resolved by increased financial participation from the French state in the functioning of the institute.

This fact stressed the separation of the two main branches: research and serological production. As a general phenomenon worldwide, pharmaceuticals, sera, and vaccines were taken over by large industrial groups who constituted a powerful industrial and economic force after World War Two. A series of national institutes in many countries meant the end of the hegemony of the Pasteur Institute and strong competition in many research fields.

Robert Koch-Institut in Berlin

The Robert Koch Institute was founded in 1891 by Robert Koch, the German bacteriologist who established the idea of specificity in the relation between infectious microbe and a particular disease.[13] He stated the bacterial cause of tuberculosis and cholera, and pioneered many fundamental bacteriological techniques. His prestige in the founding years of bacteriology makes him a sort of German *alter ego* to the figure of Louis Pasteur in France. He also became a very influential international figure. Koch first described the tuberculosis bacillus and was awarded the Nobel Prize for Medicine in 1905. Another discovery is intimately connected with the name of Robert Koch. In 1884, during a research expedition to Calcutta, India, he showed that cholera was caused by bacteria which spread through contaminated water. When cholera first broke out in Hamburg in 1892, Koch took part in the sanitary campaign. He discovered that poor drinking water treatment had led to the spread of the cholera germ. This campaign demonstrated to what extent bacteriological research and public health intervention were two sides of the same coin and the need for political intervention.

When Robert Koch first came to Berlin in 1880, he worked for the *Kaiserlichen Gesundheitsam* [Imperial Health Office]. The office had been founded in 1876, and was not initially well equipped. Facilities were improved in 1879 with better chemical and hygiene laboratories. Koch's first staff members in the new bacteriological laboratory were Georg Gaffky and Friedrich Loeffler. They both followed in his footsteps when he became director of the Institute of Infectious Diseases.

Due to his international prestige and his huge political influence, he succeeded in establishing a bacteriological research unit at the *Königlich Preussischen Instituts für Infektionskrankheiten* [Royal Prussian Institute of Infectious Diseases]. Koch was the director until 1904. In 1945 the Robert Koch Institute was merged with the *Reichsanstalt für Wasser, Boden und Lufthygiene* [Imperial Institute for Water, Soil and Air Hygiene] and the *Reichsgesundheitsamt* [Imperial Health Office] and became the *Zentralinstitut für Hygiene und Gesundheitsdienst* [Central Institute for Hygiene and Healthcare].

Although the establishment of an independent institute for the research and control of infectious diseases had been under consideration since 1887, it was not until the Tenth International Medical Conference (Berlin, 1890) that the project was implemented. Since its inauguration in July 1891, the Robert Koch Institute took over tasks for public health policies and social medicine in various municipalities. International inquiries were also answered, mostly giving expert opinions based on experimental work. The first location was next to the Charité Hospital, the largest and oldest hospital in Berlin. The scientific department was set up in a converted building known as 'The Triangle'. The institute was located in barracks on the Charité site. This solution was considered provisional, not least because an expansion of the Charité was already planned with new and functional buildings.

In 1897 the cornerstone ceremony was held for its definitive location at Nordufer, on the north-western edge of the city of Berlin. The construction work was completed in the summer of 1900. There were sheds for large and small animals for research experiments (such as cattle, horses, sheep, and even ferrets, and frogs). Simultaneously, a new city hospital was built just on the other side of the street. It opened in 1906 as the Rudolf Virchow Hospital. A specialist infections department was established at the hospital, led by a doctor who was also a staff member of the Robert Koch Institute. The principle of combining scientific research and clinical departments was successfully retained. During the following years, the institute grew continuously and new departments included a rabies protection section.[14]

The institute was named Robert Koch in 1912 to commemorate the 30th anniversary of the identification of the tuberculosis bacillus. After World War One the appellative *Königlich* [Royal] disappeared and it was renamed as 'Prussian Institute for Infectious Diseases, Robert Koch'. In 1935 the Robert Koch Institute was incorporated as a department into the *Reich Gesundheitsam* [Imperial Health Office]. Given its central position in public health administration between 1935 and 1942, being a part of the *Reich Gesundheitsam*, the institute was heavily involved in Nazi social hygiene policies and sanitary activities, but in 1942 it became an independent *Reich* body, the 'Robert Koch Institute'.[15]

In 1885, shortly after the cholera expedition to India, Koch had become professor of hygiene at the Friedrich Wilhelm University in Berlin. Prominent scientists worked in his team, among them the later nobel laureates Emil von Behring and Paul Ehrlich. Nevertheless, bacteriological evidence was not found for many infectious diseases such as smallpox or measles, and Koch admitted in the early 1890s that he had no idea of 'what kind of pathogens could be the cause'. It was not until the turn of the century that a second microbiological breakthrough occurred and a previously unknown type of pathogen was described: viruses. Tangible evidence of their existence was first found in animals. Two former pupils of Robert Koch, Friedrich Loeffler and Paul Frosch, discovered that the lymph fluid of animals with foot-and-mouth disease remained infectious even if it had previously been cleaned with a special bacterial filter. Loeffler and Frosch suspected that the cause of the unexplained infections such as smallpox, influenza, or measles, could be the very smallest pathogens, *filterable viruses,* an assumption that would later be proved true.

However, the indications for the viral pathogens remained indirect for some time. They only become visible in the 1930s, after the development of the electron microscope. An emerging branch of infection medicine – virology – became one of the most important research fields of the twentieth century at the Robert Koch Institute.

In addition to bacteria and viruses, even in the time of Robert Koch, a third type of pathogen became the focus of attention: parasites. These were associated with serious infectious diseases including malaria and sleeping sickness (an infection transmitted through tsetse flies in Africa that infects the brain). A devastating sleeping sickness epidemic raged in Congo and around Lake Victoria at the turn of the century. The German colonial areas were also affected. Robert Koch headed an expedition in 1906 on behalf of the imperial government with a team of scientists to German East Africa to investigate therapeutic options. Koch used a chemical arsenic compound called *atoxyl,* a pharmaceutical that became the standard treatment for sleeping sickness during the first decades of the twentieth century. Nevertheless, it became evident that *atoxyl* only temporarily stopped the parasites and did not heal. Koch doubled the dose with evident risk for the patients and many patients experienced severe intestinal pain, and in some cases even blindness. The colonies were an open field for human research without restrictions.

After returning to Berlin at the end of 1907, he proposed that the *Reichsgesundheitsrat* set up special isolation and treatment facilities for affected patients and to consistently use the substance to contain the spread of the disease, a strategy that was also advocated by British experts in tropical medicine. Koch's last African expedition to find a solution for trypanosomiasis (sleeping sickness) was his most unsuccessful colonial experience. He died only two and a half years later in May 1910.

After Koch's death, several smallpox epidemics affected the German population between 1916 and 1920. In addition, it turned out that the smallpox vaccine sometimes caused dangerous brain inflammation. Other outbreaks, such as the diphtheria outbreak in the early 1930s, were forcing the researchers to act quickly. Like the Pasteur Institute, the Robert Koch laboratories succeeded in improving the available vaccination procedures and protecting numerous children from diphtheria in most affected areas.

Particularly difficult for the work of the institute, however, were the political changes during the Nazi period.[16] Shortly after the Nazi seizure of power in 1933, Jewish employees were fired and had to emigrate. As a consequence of its central position in the German healthcare system, the institute was deeply involved in Nazi violence. Some of its employees were involved in human clinical trials in concentration camps. Towards the end of World War Two, the activities of the institute could only be continued to a limited extent due to bomb damage, personnel shortages, and material deficiencies. After the war, the remaining employees initially worked under difficult conditions. In 1952 the institute became part of the newly founded *Bundesgesundheitsamts* [Federal Health Office], but it was not until the 1960s that the researchers again enjoyed modern facilities and rooms.

An important aspect of the institute was the attention devoted to technical facilities. Microscopy had always played a central role in the research on infectious diseases. The Ernst Leitz optical works were one of the world's most successful microscope manufacturers at the beginning of the twentieth century. In 1907, they built their 100,000th piece and handed it to Robert Koch. His research on anthrax experiments achieved a milestone when he could observe the pathogen material in infected animals and then transmitted the disease to mice, which he had previously infected with anthrax. Koch observed that the infection was triggered by some sort of chain-forming bacteria. He also saw punctate structures in the anthrax bacteria – the so-called spores – when he observed them in dried preparations and recognised that only spore-containing material was capable of being infected. He drew these observations carefully and used microphotography as one of the best procedures for representing the results objectively.[17]

In the late nineteenth century, various technical developments were quickly driving the field of bacteriological and serological research. Microscopy was one of them. The physicist Ernst Abbe developed lenses with such a high resolution that, for example, mycobacteria, including the causative agent of tuberculosis, could be observed. Just as important was Robert Koch's discovery of the so-called *Reink Cultures*: the targeted cultivation of bacterial colonies in culture media. Microscopy and dyeing, together with tissue cultivation techniques, enabled the isolation of pathogens from animal and human material and the ability to transmit the infection to other animals. This development was boosted by colonial social medicine policies: workers and soldiers in the colonies were affected by a wide range of tropical diseases that were susceptible to experimental research in the laboratory. There was a need for research in the field, and the state was prepared to invest large sums. Simultaneously, microscopes and other laboratory technologies improved and so technical demands for better research were soon implemented.

Nevertheless, there were other pathogens so tiny that they escaped the best light microscopes: viruses. Only several decades later, in 1931, did engineers Bodo von Borries and Ernst Ruska built the first electron microscope in Berlin. It achieved a significantly higher resolution than light microscopes. Ten years later, the Robert Koch Institute received the first device as a donation from the AEG Company (German industry was very strong in the manufacture of laboratory instruments at the time). Electron microscopy constituted a transcendental technical background for future contributions from the Robert Koch Institute and an exhibition of technological power. In the early phase of microbiologic research, microscopy was used to detect pathogens and researchers focused on its use following outbreaks, or for studying biological hazards.

At the end of World War Two, the Robert Koch Institute was assigned – with the approval of the allied powers – to the health administration of the city of Berlin. From June 1945 onwards, the institute was given the task of controlling epidemics by the magistrate of the City of Berlin following corresponding orders from the Soviet occupying power. The institute became part of the *Bundes Gesundheits Amt* (Federal Health Office) in 1952 and retained this status until the dissolution of the office in 1994. Since then the Robert Koch Institute has been an independent federal institute with a large department responsible for health reporting and epidemiology.

London School of Hygiene and Tropical Medicine and national research institutes in Britain

Britain developed an interest in tropical diseases when infections, plagues, and contagions affecting the colonies became a matter of concern and a field of research from the perspective of new bacteriological methods. Moreover, the emphasis was directed towards the prevention of diseases affecting British travellers, while the indigenous population in colonial tropical countries were also the target. Initially, the foundation of the *London School of Hygiene and Tropical Medicine* was closely linked to healthcare provision for seamen returning from the colonies.[18] Sailors represented a large social group from the healthcare perspective in the context of the British Empire, and establishments were founded for this purpose from the first decades of the nineteenth century. A Seamen's Hospital Society was founded by public voluntary subscriptions in 1821 for establishing a floating hospital. It was devoted to the assistance and relief of sick and helpless seamen. Patients were treated on ships moored on the Thames. New facilities were moved to land in 1870 as a part of Greenwich Hospital, and in 1890 the Seamen's Hospital Society opened a branch hospital at the Royal Albert Dock.[19] In short, tropical medicine started in London as a clinical discipline (endowed with a bacteriological, serological, and parasitological input) that was closely linked to health problems in the colonies.

In addition, as the colonies were the main focus of infectious diseases, research led by the institution in London appeared as an opportunity for advancement in this field. The sanitary staff during the first decades of hospital care were doctors and nurses with practical professional experience in the colonies.[20] The care of civil and military servants of the British Empire, as well as the training of medical officers was a major activity. The school was founded by Patrick Manson, a doctor who had worked in the Far East from the 1860s to the 1880s, where he became aware of the importance of research on tropical diseases. He returned to London and began work at St George's Hospital in 1892. His work with seamen suffering from tropical diseases helped to convince the medical authorities that training in this area was necessary. Similarly, Ronald Ross (1857–1932) was working as a doctor in the Indian Medical Service when he did research associating the transmission of malaria with the Anopheles mosquito (1897). For this discovery, which opened new expectations in the fight against the disease, he was awarded the Nobel Prize for Medicine in 1902.

The huge importance of tropical medicine and experimental research in the colonies was assumed by the health authorities. Consequently, a School for Tropical Medicine opened its doors in 1899, starting with the modest figure of 11 students. The school was a part of the Seamen's Hospital Society's Branch Hospital at the Albert Dock. The object of the school was to acquaint students with tropical diseases and teach therapeutic procedures, as well as to train staff in research methods, observe, record, and discover new procedures for fighting infectious disease.

The initiative was a success. After the first five years of teaching, the London School of Tropical Medicine (1899–1904) had instructed 564 students. They were mostly young men, but 36 women also received instruction.[21] All students had some sanitary qualification before attending the course at the school, and students went on to work in missions and hospitals overseas to fulfil practical training periods. In the case of malaria, several students were sent to the Roman Campagna near the mouth of River Tiber in Italy to carry out experiments on the prevention of malaria. They spent three months from June to October living in a wooden hut in the malaria infested region. By staying inside the hut from dusk until dawn they all escaped infection. After the malaria hut experiment some researchers went to the West Indies to study *filariasis*. It was in the context of these practical training activities that G.C. Low demonstrated the passage of *filariae* in the mosquito proboscis and its entry into the human host via the bite.[22] The expedition was extended at the request of Patrick Manson who proposed that visits should be made to other West Indian islands, such as Barbados (where the rate of affected patients was high), and Grenada (where it was low) in order to compare and contrast the circumstances of the islands. These research programmes aimed to throw light on the conditions that favoured the infection. Patrick Manson also conducted an experiment to obtain evidence on the transmission of malaria in humans by mosquitoes (1900). Volunteers, including his son, were bitten by infected mosquitoes and developed malaria. The volunteers were quickly treated with quinine and recovered from the disease. The outcome of the experiment was a fundamental demonstration of the mosquito-malaria theory.

Another prominent foundational figure was Francis Lovell, who had worked all over the world in his early career – including a position as chief medical officer and president of the General Board of Health in Mauritius, and surgeon-general of Trinidad and Tobago until his retirement from the Colonial Medical Service in 1901. Back in London, he became involved in raising funds for the school and was elected Dean in 1903. The school also recruited Aldo Castellani to join a sleeping sickness commission in Uganda, where he researched the disease in 1902. In 1903, Castellani described trypanosomes in the cerebral fluid of a patient suffering from sleeping sickness. He suspected a bacterial cause and so did not realise the importance of his finding. Meanwhile, David Bruce recognised the significance of the discovery, which led to the controversy over priority. Castellani was an active participant in the League of Nations Health Organisation activities, helped to establish the Ross Institute in 1926, and later became the Director of Mycology at the London School of Hygiene and Tropical Medicine.

Parasitology was also a prominent research field at the London School. Robert Leiper focused his research on helminthology, the study of parasitic worms. He spent his early career travelling to Egypt, Uganda, the Gold Coast, China, and Japan, making essential contributions to the knowledge of the life cycles of many helminths. He actively participated in establishing the new School of Hygiene & Tropical Medicine in 1924 and worked at the school until his retirement in 1947. Another researcher was William Simpson, who lectured at the school from its opening in 1899 until he retired in 1923, being also professor of Hygiene at King's College, London. As most of his colleagues working on tropical medicine, in addition to his academic work, he travelled extensively, often at the request of the government to deal with outbreaks of plague, enteric fever, dysentery, and other public health problems in the colonies. Between 1923 and 1926 Simpson worked with Castellani to establish the Ross Institute in Putney.

Popularisation of hygiene occupied an important place among the activities of the school. Hugh Newham attended the school in 1906 as a student. He then became demonstrator and succeeded C.W. Daniels as director and superintendent in 1910. He worked for the British Military Health Administration as a consultant in tropical diseases during World War One. On his return to the school, he was tasked with organising the museum and teaching collections until his retirement in 1938. During this period, public health museums were the main instruments for teaching health education to the general public.

Wickliffe Rose, director of the Rockefeller Foundation International Health Board, visited Robert Leiper at the London School for consultation on hookworm disease. The Rockefeller funded national campaigns in many countries that were focused on this professional illness that affected miners worldwide.[23] This meeting marked the start of a long and fruitful connection between the London School and the Rockefeller Foundation – which after the war would convert the initial school into the London School of Hygiene & Tropical Medicine.

Following the outbreak of war in 1914, many members of staff were called for service overseas. Student numbers also fell dramatically from 1914 to 1918. Thereafter, the end of the war offered the school new perspectives and opportunities and it was felt that the war would create an increase in patients suffering from tropical diseases in England. Indeed, the war produced a dramatic sanitary catastrophe in the post-war years. As health services worldwide came under increasing pressure, politicians came to understand the benefits of international surveillance and cooperation. This was also the logical reaction to the devastating post-war worldwide influenza pandemic of 1918 and 1919, as well as huge famines in numerous territories, and local epidemic outbreaks of typhus, famine, venereal diseases, and tuberculosis.[24] Acknowledging the organisational and financial confusion caused by healthcare being fragmented between different departments, the British government set up the Ministry of Health in 1919. This was created as a reconstruction of the Local Government Board.

The school and the *Hospital for Tropical Diseases* moved to Endsleigh Gardens in central London in 1920, taking over a former hotel that had been used as a hospital for officers during the war. The first cases were patients affected by bilharziasis, malaria, amoebic and bacillary dysentery, liver abscess, kala-azar, sleeping sickness (*trypanosomiase*) and other tropical diseases. With the new challenges identified after the war, the LSHTM received a new impulse. In 1921 the Post-Graduate Medical Committee chaired by Lord Athlone recommended a new orientation, which was established under the influence of the Rockefeller Foundation. It consisted of the establishment of an Institute of Medicine in association with the London University, as a postgraduate centre for teaching and research in public health.[25] The Trustees of the Rockefeller Foundation made this recommendation possible by giving two million dollars towards the establishment of the school, and the British government undertook to provide a grant of £25,000 a year towards the upkeep of the school for the first five years.

Andrew Balfour was appointed director of the Wellcome Tropical Research Laboratories in Khartoum and local Medical Officer of Health during the period

1902–1913. He worked closely with the League of Nations as a member of several expert bodies and a delegate of the British administration.[26] In addition, negotiations were opened with other bodies operating in the same sphere for cooperation with the new school.[27] Balfour returned to London to found and direct the Wellcome Bureau of Scientific Research. He undertook important work in several countries during the First World War (including Egypt, Iraq, Tanganyika and Palestine), and became the first director of the new London School of Hygiene & Tropical Medicine in 1924. In his presidential address to the Royal Society of Tropical Medicine and Hygiene (1925), Balfour called for a balance between preventive public health and clinical medicine.[28]

In accordance with internal documents, the new institute was intended to help the government maintain standards of health and grow enough crops to feed the population after the war. The Ministry of Agriculture agreed to fund a study of parasites affecting farm animals and plants. With further funding, Leiper was able to pursue a second strand of research in comparative parasitology.

The Empire Marketing Board approved a grant for research into the technique of milk examination in 1931. This research was conducted by Graham Wilson, an expert in bacteriology applied to hygiene at LSHTM. In 1934, the Minister of Health and the Minister of Agriculture received a deputation of researchers from LSHTM to discuss ensuring a clean and safe milk supply for the country. The deputation urged compulsory pasteurisation, eradication of disease in cattle, and the stimulation of clean milk production.

At the outbreak of World War One, it was decided that the school office would remain in Keppel Street as long as possible, despite an offer of accommodation made by Queen's College in Cambridge. During the war, staff and student numbers were drastically reduced and space was offered to other organisations, and for the training of military personnel. Some of the school's vaults were used as public air-raid shelters throughout the war.

The school was initially managed by a governing body but it received a Royal Charter that enabled incorporation with a board of management and a court of governors composed of 34 members. Three of the governors were appointed by the Ministry of Health, three by the senate of the University of London, two by the Seamen's Hospital Society, six by the General Medical Council, and one board member was appointed by each of the Secretaries of State of Home Affairs, Colonies, India, Air, and War – as well as the Admiralty, and the president of Board of Education. Other members were appointed by the Minister of Agriculture and Fisheries, the Secretary for Scotland, the Medical Research Council, the Health Committee of the League of Nations, London County Council, County Councils Association, Municipal Corporations Association, Lister Institute, British Medical Association, Society of Medical Officers of Health, Royal Sanitary Institute, and the Royal Institute of Public Health.[29] This long list of governors indicates to what extent the renewed institution had a state, national, and international vocation.

The provisional management and supervisory body of the school was based on a transitional executive committee consisting of nine persons, three of them appointed by the Court of Governors, three by the Minister of Health, two by the

Senate of the University of London and one by the Seamen's Hospital Society. The board made statutes for the school's regulation and management.

The British Ministry of Health sent in 1925 a memorandum to the League of Nations on the organisation and functions of the Ministry of Health.[30] The official report stated that one of the functions of the Ministry of Health was to lead research in public health and social medicine. For this purpose, it maintained three laboratories: a Bacteriological Laboratory, the Government Lymph Establishment (for the preparation of vaccine lymph), and a Foods (Chemical) Laboratory. Special arrangements were made for experimental research on cases of food poisoning. Medical officers of the Ministry of Health had undertaken several enquiries into health problems relating to cancer, influenza, rheumatism, tuberculosis, and lethargic encephalitis.

The Medical Research Council was established out of the Ministry of Health under the Ministry of Health Act. The general principles guiding research were specified as: (a) dealing with problems of immediate practical interest arising from current administration; and (b) dealing with enquiries necessitating local enquiries or collaboration with local authorities, and the council with problems involving more extended investigation than those under or arising independently of immediate administrative needs.[31]

There was no general public service statistical department in Britain. The Minister of Health was responsible for the compilation of statistics including the administration of the sale of Food and Drugs Act and national health insurance. Statistical enquiries were also carried out under the direction of the Medical Research Council together with Ministry of Health and other government departments.

Social medicine and sanitary policies in Hungary

Public health started its institutionalisation in Hungary at the end of the nineteenth century as in many other European countries. Joseph Fodor, a pupil of the German hygienist, Max von Pettenkofer, convinced the authorities of the insufficiency of present state healthcare and the need to establish an institute of hygiene in Budapest. Cholera epidemics in 1872 and 1873 prompted the creation of a chair of hygiene (1874) – subsequently occupied by Fodor. Initially the new institute was established as a part of the Institute of Physiology. Physiology and hygiene shared academic space in most European countries. By 1909, the institute included a laboratory and an office for the professor, an assistant's laboratory, and another laboratory for trainees, a room for work on physics and chemistry, a small work room, a small space for the laboratory assistant, a small darkroom for photography, and a library. It did not have a lecture room and teaching took place in the amphitheatre of the Institute of Physiology. From this initiative, the teaching of public health started its institutionalisation. This chapter discusses the schools of hygiene and training conditions of public health officers in Hungary.[32]

Hungary took steps in public health policies after World War One. In November 1925, Selskar M. Gunn, director of the International Health Board of the Rockefeller Foundation, and the delegate of its Paris office, wrote a letter to

Norman White, a member of the Health Section of the League of Nations, reporting the development of health reforms in Hungary. From his words, it is easy to assess the huge influence of transnational organisations on national initiatives and the network of participants intervening in the process.[33]

> When I was in Hungary recently, I had some conversations with Dr. Scholtz, the Under-Secretary of State for Health in the Ministry of Public Welfare, with regard to the relationship of the Hungarian public health authorities and the Health Section of the League of Nations. I had a definite impression that there exists some slight misunderstanding on the part of the Hungarians with regard to the whole question. I believe there has been some correspondence between Rajchmann and the health authorities, and I have an idea that the Hungarian health authorities are perhaps waiting for some kind of action on the part of the Health Section.
>
> As you may know, there has been created in Budapest a Sanitary Reform Bureau, which is connected with the Ministry of Public Welfare (this Ministry includes all public health activities). It has been practically decided that this Sanitary Reform Bureau will act as liaison bureau with the Health Section of the League of Nations. It seemed to the Hungarians, and I think they are right, that it was not necessary to set up an entirely separate bureau for the purpose of being in relation with the Health Section of the League, and that the Sanitary Reform Bureau could very readily take care of this. The Sanitary Reform Bureau has some very capable young men most of whom have had the benefit of travel trips in America and elsewhere.
>
> Dr Kornel Scholtz, who recently took the place of Dr Fay, is an unusually good man, very easy to cooperate with and has a broad point of view.
>
> The Sanitary Reform Bureau is already doing quite a lot of work, some of which I think might be of interest. For example, Dr B. Johan,[34] who is director of the new Institute of Hygiene, which is now being built in Budapest, is making special statistical studies in connection with cancer. Johan is one of the outstanding public health men in Central Europe, an excellently trained doctor, with broad public health knowledge, speaking French, English, and German very well. I think it would be a very good idea, if possible, to have the Health Section of the League of Nations invite Dr Scholtz or Dr Johan to go to Geneva for a short time. I do not mean on the permanent staff, but simply to pay a short visit, such as that made by Dr Kuhn, or Dr Stampar's staff.[35] If this invitation could be arranged from your end, I feel sure that if it were necessary I could find the funds to finance the trip.[36]

Gunn's report to Norman White aimed to express that there existed in Hungary in 1925 a very definite desire on the part of the public health authorities to be in closer relation with the Health Section and Committee of the League of Nations. Gunn expressed literally the positive advantages derived from international cooperation and bringing the Hungarians within the group of countries under the influence of the League and the Rockefeller Foundation. Gunn insisted on the opportunity of opening formal relations between the League of Nations and Hungary, proposing a letter of invitation to Kornel Scholtz to visit the League. He showed a huge interest in integrating Hungary as a preferential country for sanitary reforms supported by the League.

Gunn's confidential report to White gave not only information about the initiatives in Hungary, but also shows the transnational networks moving the threads of public health initiatives in Europe. Those expert lobbies managed expertise and political initiatives. In the next chapter, we shall refer to the instruction of public health experts in Poland.

National Institute of Hygiene and Public Health in Poland

In February 1917, the Polish government instituted a section for public health under the leadership of Witold Chodzko, a psychiatrist and delegate for public health affairs at the League of Nations. He was very active in the process of institutionalisation and transnational cooperation, to the extent that he became one of the most prominent participants in the international scene. The initial section in Warsaw grew and finally became a ministry in 1918, a month after the signing of the German-Russian peace treaty.[37]

The huge health problems affecting the Polish population at the end of World War One, were impossible to challenge from a purely national perspective. Poland suffered one of the greatest material destructions among European countries during the war. M.A. Balinska states that around one third of the 27 million Poles were seriously undernourished and the country had a huge number of refugees, which naturally favoured the spread of contagious diseases such as dysentery, relapsing fever, smallpox, sexually transmitted diseases, tuberculosis, and most spectacularly typhus, which soon evolved into a pandemic affecting Russia, the Ukraine, and eastern regions of Poland.[38] Reliable sources estimated that there were probably around 25 to 30 million cases of typhus in the transnational region between 1919 and 1921. Around four million cases were reported in Poland, with some three million deaths due to infectious diseases after the war. Foreign relief agencies provided valuable assistance, with one of the most remarkable efforts being made by the *American Relief Administration* (ARA), which helped primarily with feeding programmes for children. The agency worked together with the Polish Committee for Aid to Children (*Polski Komitet Pomocy Dzieciom*).[39]

To respond to the sanitary emergency, the National Epidemiological Institute was established in Warsaw in November 1918 to act as a governmental agency centralising epidemiological intelligence, diagnosis of cases and prevention, notably by means of an effort for vaccine and sera production. The institute also coordinated anti-epidemic measures, which were necessary due to the lack of health personnel. Most practitioners were victims of the war and there were civil disturbances throughout the nation.

The Epidemiological Institute later became a National Institute of Hygiene. It was supported by the work of Ludwik Rajchman, who worked as an activist in the internationalisation of public health policies, mainly as a bridge between the Rockefeller Foundation and the League of Nations.[40] Rajchman was strongly supported in his efforts by Poland's first two ministers of health, Witold Chodzko and Tomasz Janiszewski, both active members in Polish initiatives on health policies and in transnational actions with the League of Nations Health Committee and Organisation. These ministers acted as a powerful lobby. The frightening outbreak of epidemics just after the war gave urgency to the inauguration of the institute in spring 1919.

The severity of the health situation was brought to international attention through the alarming reports of the Polish authorities and Western relief organisations. Polish appeals to the League of Nations early in 1920 resulted in the designation of an International Epidemic Commission to which the director of the Central Epidemiological Institute and head of the Health Organisation of the League of Nations, Ludwik Rajchman, was appointed commissioner. The International Epidemic Commission established offices in Warsaw in the buildings of the institute (which was serving as an epidemiological intelligence body and supplying protective sera and vaccines, and thereby fulfilling a similar role to that of the previously mentioned national institutes of hygiene during the First World War).

Despite the difficult working conditions and scarce resources after the war, the institute laboratories increased production of serological products and vaccines 'from 862 litres in 1919 to 7,302 litres in 1920 and, after the cessation of hostilities, the institute exported part of its production to Russia and Greece, via the League of Nations'.[41] In addition, the international sanitary conference held in Warsaw in March 1922, convened by the League of Nations, opened the doors for the League to be entrusted with the coordination of international health and anti-epidemic measures for all of Eastern Europe.[42]

Once more the Rockefeller Foundation was an essential supporter for the establishment of the National Institute of Hygiene. Rajchman and Chozko were very active, playing prominent roles in the international sanitary actions promoted by the League of Nations. After the Warsaw Conference (1922) the Polish government and the Rockefeller Foundation started discussions on public health issues. Wickliffe Rose, a bacteriologist and head of the International Health Board, attended the conference.[43] Rajchman was the principal mediator among leaders from Poland and the Rockefeller Foundation. He was well acquainted with the French and British laboratories and therefore worked to introduce research activities at the Polish Institute and for the establishment of a National School of Hygiene as essential tools for professionalisation. This was also RF policy in Hungary, Czechoslovakia, Yugoslavia, and Spain. The training policy for public health experts was also similar: a series of fellowships were offered for a limited number of specialists, who were to assume key positions in the health administration on their return to Poland.

Although Poland went through a difficult financial situation after the war and suffered from political instability, the RF's International Health Board recognised that the country 'had made great progress during the last year and industries were recovering'.[44] Their favourable attitude was no doubt strengthened by the praise given to the Polish health authorities by Colonel Gilchrist, who had worked with the Central Epidemiological Institute and the high esteem in which Rajchman's achievements were held by the League of Nations.

Consequently, the Rockefeller Foundation contributed $215,000 towards the building of a National School of Hygiene.[45] In addition, the American Jewish Joint Distribution Committee donated $40,000. Rajchman was Jewish and the committee created a specialist board for public health in Poland, whose head was Bernard Flexner, brother of the then director of the Rockefeller Institute. Wickliffe Rose mediated for his involvement.[46]

The institute hosted the national school, as well as three other divisions: (a) production of sera and vaccine; (b) chemistry; and (c) bacteriology, protozoology and experimental medicine. The former Central Epidemiological Institute became a national hygiene institute in 1923 and whose main functions were initially 'diagnosis of infectious diseases, research of their nature, routes of transmission, methods of control, as well as the production and experimental studies of sera, vaccines, and other bacteriological products'.[47] The institute's role was broadened in 1927 to 'research on public hygiene to meet the needs of public health'.[48]

The RF was mainly involved in the project for a school of hygiene directed by Witold Chodzko. However, the RF also supported certain research programmes linked to the department of physiological chemistry and nutrition. Rajchman influenced this orientation to develop studies on dietary habits and deficiency diseases after his visits to the Johns Hopkins and Harvard Schools of Public Health.[49] To lead this new research, Kazimierz Funk was appointed after his prominent contributions to research on vitamins. Following a grant of $3,600 from the RF and with technical equipment obtained from Germany, Austria, and Czechoslovakia, Funk led Poland to become an entirely self-sufficient producer and later exporter of insulin – and only the third European country to manufacture the hormone.

As in Prague and Madrid, the RF was interested in the establishment of a model of healthcare centre linked to the National Institute of Hygiene (NIH) to serve as pattern for healthcare reform. A new health centre at Mokotow was developed as a model and was visited by health officers from around the country to receive instruction about organisation and programmes. The initiative consisted in establishing about 500 similar centres throughout Poland during the following 15 years.[50] The centre included a disinfection unit and an experimental sewage station. At the time, the treatment of sewage was essential for agricultural and medical reasons and the RF supported the plan, considering that the Warsaw model could serve as a teaching centre for sanitary engineers and chemists from other central and eastern European countries. The RF also showed interest in the establishment of an Institute of Mental Health, which was finally established in 1935, a critical period when the great depression affected the economy and reduced the funds for programmes at the National Institute of Hygiene.

The Warsaw Institute represents the concept of a state institution coordinating and implementing public health policies. From the outset, it established a network of centres in major towns. International influence was evident at personal and institutional levels. Rajchman contributed his experiences at the Pasteur Institute and the Medical Research Council when setting up the Central Epidemiological Institute for the production and trade of sera and vaccines. Similarly, the structure, purposes, and programmes were similar to those enacted by other European institutes.

In less than two decades, the Warsaw NIH managed to build up departments of bacteriology and experimental medicine, sera and vaccines, chemistry, food and consumer goods, water, and an institute of mental hygiene. Bacteriological analyses for the control of contagious diseases were carried out by the NIH and its subsidiaries; quality control for food and other goods had been unified into a single system; most sewers were systematically tested by the institute, and the entire national and international production of sera and vaccines was controlled by the NIH before being marketed.[51] In terms of the output of biological products, the institute was entirely self-sufficient and received no help from the government. Nevertheless, the institute experienced a deep crisis during World War Two and the post-war years.

Central Institute of Hygiene in Belgrade

The project of establishing an institute for public health to research infectious diseases and produce sera and vaccines in Belgrade started immediately after the First World War. An Institute of Public Health of Belgrade was initially established in 1919, when a ministerial commission for epidemiology was organised by the Ministry of Health to monitor communicable diseases and alleviate the negative consequences of the war. Milan Jovanovic Batut was the first head of the commission, but the new institution lacked sufficient financial support and technical expertise. This was the first step for the establishment of a Central Institute of Hygiene in Belgrade a few years later. The project was widely discussed and finally on 25 October 1924, the new institution was established by a decree of the Yugoslavian government.[52] The final decision was decisively implemented thanks to the intervention of the Croat Andrija Stampar in the negotiations with the Rockefeller Foundation.[53] The institute became the site of the entire health institution administration, including a national hygiene service. The director was appointed by the Ministry of Public Health. The Central Hygiene Institute received the second largest Rockefeller grant in Yugoslavia, after the School of Public Health in Zagreb, led by Stampar. This represented a balance for the tense rivalry between the two capital cities.[54]

The internal reports of the Rockefeller Foundation state that the institute was conceived to coordinate epidemiological initiatives and bacteriological laboratories in Yugoslavia for controlling plagues and infectious diseases. In addition, it provided experimental support to public health campaigns, producing sera and vaccines, while regulating the consumption and trade of these products inside the country. Moreover, the Central Hygiene Institute taught public health experts and participated in health education campaigns. Before closing the agreement, the Rockefeller Foundation requested from S. Miletic, minister of public health, his commitment to adapt the Belgrade institution to other national institutes in Europe supported by the Rockefeller Foundation. After negotiations with Stampar and Miletic, the International Health Board of the RF approved in 1925 a grant of $30,000 for equipping the Institute, a budget subject to the supervision of A. Stampar. The RF was consulted regarding the best profile for the future director of the institute and Stevan Ivanic was subsequently appointed.

The Central Hygiene Institute of Belgrade started work in 1926. It integrated three institutions previously founded in 1922: the Permanent Bacteriological Station, the Institute of Social Medicine, and the Institute for Tropical Diseases. The new institution included nine sections: diagnosis; sera and vaccines; water improvement, containing several sections for bacteriology, biochemistry and chemistry, zoology and health technologies; control of foodstuffs; parasitology; epidemiology; serology; pedagogy and propaganda; and hospitalisation. All these sections were organised in three large departments: bacteriological-epidemiological; chemical; and parasitological, sanitary engineering and socio-medical.[55] In general it reproduced the standard structure of national institutes of hygiene in Europe, independently of small peculiarities and differences. Each section had a simple structure. It was led by a head of section and had technical and administrative staff in accordance with the budget available. The Central Institute was the instrument of the state for the implementation of experimental research and public health policies.

The institute also encompassed various socio-medical centres located in Belgrade and its surroundings, such as the Hospital for Infectious Diseases, the Institute for the Protection of Mothers and Children, the Museum of Hygiene, the Polyclinic School, the Institute for Research and Control of Cancer, among other agencies.

Besides the Central Institute of Hygiene there was an Institute for Tropical Diseases at Skopje. Formally, the institute was conceived as an external department of the Central Hygiene Institute in Belgrade, although in practical terms it enjoyed absolute independence. It coordinated all the institutions and programmes related with research and control of tropical diseases – mostly malaria. All national institutions working on tropical diseases reported to the institute and a director was responsible for its management. The Skopje Institute contained four sections: serology and bacteriology; chemistry; parasitology; malaria and same origin diseases.

Due to its very active research and social work, the Skopje Institute soon attracted the attention of the Rockefeller International Health Board. To further develop the network of centres devoted to social medicine in Macedonia under the coordination of the Skopje Institute, the RF supported the establishment of small health stations (staffed with a nurse, a sanitary inspector, and an assistant) in the most impoverished rural districts that lacked any healthcare service. Around 50 of those very small rural healthcare centres were planned. The pattern was similar in other European countries, such as Poland, Bulgaria, Spain, and Czechoslovakia.

After World War Two, all of this organisation collapsed. A new state introduced deep reforms in 1945. The Federal Institute of Hygiene, the Institute of Epidemiology, and the Institute of Bacteriology and Epidemiology of the Republic of Serbia were established under the guidelines of the Central Institute of Hygiene.

Prague as a social hygiene laboratory

During the first decades of the twentieth century Czechoslovak hygienists and health officials pressured for the modernisation of healthcare centres and social services.[56] The previous Imperial Health Act published in 1870 was similar to other poor and charity legislation found in many European nations, and represented an initial step in liberal reformism. The new-born Czechoslovak Republic had to face post-war reconstruction, housing shortages, famine, and very poor epidemiological conditions.

Health policies were coordinated by a Ministry of Health and Physical Training in the early 1920s, but it suffered from a lack of financial resources for modernising the old healthcare model. Moreover, there was a resistance by medical professionals to losing their self-employed status and they opposed state intervention.[57] Thanks to voluntary welfare organisations, ambulatory surgeries existed throughout the country, and health and social care houses and national health institutions were established. Their number increased considerably and over 1000 mother and children clinics, nearly 200 dispensaries for tuberculosis patients, and about 30 clinics for sexually transmitted diseases were established after World War One.[58] This was the governmental response to the main sanitary problems, a common locus in most European countries.

American post-war relief, national and international charitable missions, and especially the Rockefeller Foundation, facilitated the construction of the State Health Institute which opened in Prague in 1925. But institutional growth could only be effective with efficient expertise, and therefore the RF also developed a system of grants for Czech hygienists. The Rockefeller Foundation grantees went to Johns Hopkins to learn experimental and clinical research, epidemiology, statistics, and applied methods of biological and social sciences.

Initiatives to modernise healthcare facilities by establishing a new model of primary healthcare centre started at the end of the First World War. District healthcare centres, social care houses, and national health institutions arose thanks to the work of the American and Czechoslovak Red Cross, the Masaryk League against Tuberculosis, Care for Youth, Protection of Mothers and Children, Our Children, and other associations.[59] Most organisations were managed by committees of trustees composed of state representatives, medical experts, and delegates of the associations involved.

The 'model district' in the 13th district of Prague was an example of a new institution providing both curative and preventive healthcare. Prague had become the Czechoslovak capital at the end of the war and a 'model district' approach – supervised by the state health institute – was used to implement new methods of healthcare and social medicine. Greater Prague was formed in 1920 by joining 38 neighbouring towns and villages. The total population reached 750,000 inhabitants under a single municipal administration.[60]

After the war, sanitary staff was scarce in the city. Nineteen municipal health inspectors and the same number of district doctors assumed responsibility for the inspection and control of all hygiene regulations. The new municipal organisation also had 14 school doctors and three dentists for children. Ladislav Prokop Procházka was chief health officer for Prague during the period 1910 to 1935. He was also minister of health after the war (1920–1921). Procházka participated in the representative bodies of the League of Nations. He proposed the reorganisation of the health service in the early 1920s by creating a health office for the City of Prague endowed with executive power under the direction of a chief medical officer. The health department of the city was changed to a health office, and included statistics, chemical, bacteriological, demographic, veterinary and market sections. The Health Commission acted as an advisory board for the central authorities of the municipality. In short, after World War One, Prague experienced a new organisation of healthcare and social medicine.

Health officers reported to the Ministry of Health and Physical Training (founded in 1918). Linked to the central health administration, these officers were central participants for implementing social hygiene policies. The health office of the City of Prague managed five town district offices, while the sixth office was the new model health district in the 13th district of Prague, directly under the chief medical officer.[61]

Procházka also established a central board of consulting rooms in collaboration with the municipality. It was endowed with post-natal, infant, and children's clinics. A series of offices and organisations were involved: the Central Social Office, Chief Medical Officers's Office, Red Cross, League against Tuberculosis, Care for Youth and others. The *model district Vršovice – Praha 13* joined the scheme and coordinated social work and health care services.[62]

At the Czech Conference of Health and Social Work (1928), plans for the next ten years were discussed and agreed. Social assistance and healthcare were assessed in several rural and urban districts. Procházka was the main driving force of the 'model district in Prague 13th'. Social assistance and healthcare centres were conceived as national institutions, maintained by a cooperation between the state administration and civil society, with the collaboration of voluntary philanthropic organisations.

The 13th district of Prague – one of the largest districts of Greater Prague with over 80,000 inhabitants – had been chosen to serve as an experimental area for *model work* in healthcare and social assistance. It had a suitable location and a long tradition of civil involvement and activism. The population was favourable to participating and the district was overcrowded with a growing population of workers, clerks, and peasants. Due to its plural composition, it combined the problems of a large city with those of rural districts. The local branch of the Czechoslovak Red Cross had built up a network of healthcare houses giving first aid, as well as health resorts for children, dentist's clinics, and foodbanks.[63]

An act passed on 12 October 1925 established a national health institute in Prague.[64] Placed under the Ministry of Health and Physical Training, it was conceived to carry out scientific work under the instructions of the state health administration, and also taught preventive medicine and health specialists. It included a central institute in Prague and branches at the higher schools specialised in various scientific lines.

The NHI in Prague was conceived to coordinate and offer help and advice on health issues to all public services and individuals. Internal regulations determined in which cases the NHI was authorised to make charges for work done. Charges and prices for manufactured preparations were fixed by the Ministry of Health and Physical Training and the Ministry of Finance. The NHI was managed by a director and an assistant-director. The rest of the staff consisted of technical officials carrying out scientific work, an accountancy department, a secretariat, and subordinate staff.

The institute had a special advisory board attached to the Ministry of Public Health, dealing with technical and scientific questions. The working programme, started in 1925 with the inauguration, included:

1   Routine laboratory service.
2   The rendering of decisions on special questions of public health importance on the request of the Ministry of Public Health, other authorities, and private persons.
3   Giving advice to health organisations on standardisation of laboratory methods in public health institutions.
4   Independent research on problems of practical importance.
5   Training of doctors for public work, public health specialists, as well as school doctors, food experts, and industrial and housing inspectors.
6   Training of auxiliary personnel, disinfectors, sanitary inspectors, and any other public health staff.

The NHI in Prague was composed of 11 departments:

Department I handled the preparation of sera and vaccines for national distribution and sale. Some biological products were specifically mentioned: bacterial vaccines, tuberculin, antigens, diagnostic and therapeutic sera, standardisation of vaccines and sera. The control and regulation of biological products was also handled.[65]

Department II was responsible for the production of smallpox vaccine.

Department III was named the Pasteur Department and focussed on the preparation of Pasteur vaccine, ambulatory treatment, shipment of Pasteur vaccine to other stations and doctors, research on rabies, and educational programmes.

Department IV developed an advisory role and also researched activities on syphilis, animal parasites, and insects important for public health. It also dealt with the collection of epidemiological data related to epidemic diseases, collections of cultures of microorganisms, as well as the standardisation and control of disinfectants. It managed training courses for public health workers, disinfectors, auxiliary public health personnel, and other related professionals. It included a section on tuberculosis, including diagnosis, preparation of vaccines, and specific training for specialists.

Department V dealt with the analysis and examination of the quality of food and the control of adulterations. It trained school medical inspectors and organised regular courses for public health officers and market supervisors.

Department VI was responsible for the examination of drugs and pharmaceuticals.

Department VII worked on nutrition and dietetics. It did research, collaborated in food quality control, researched vegetarianism and vitamins, among other issues. It also trained school medical inspectors.

Department VIII was responsible for sanitary engineering, including water supply, examination of mineral waters, water contamination, purification and disinfection of water and sewage systems, as well as the standardisation of methods. Together with other departments, it collaborated in educational activities and trained public health officers and general doctors, sanitary engineers, and auxiliary personnel, such as disinfectors and water supervisors.

Department IX focussed on housing hygiene, helped in the preparation of courses for public health officers, doctors, sanitary engineers, and social workers.

Department X dealt with school hygiene and monitored school conditions and installations. It also trained school doctors, public health workers, general doctors, teachers, school nurses, and social workers.

Department XI focussed on industrial hygiene. It supervised the sanitary conditions of factories and workshops, the health of industrial workers, and cooperated with international labour organisations. This section also reported on and issued licenses for activities related to industrial hygiene, equipment, and material conditions for workers. In addition, it gave postgraduate courses for doctors, trained industrial inspectors and public health officers, and gave lectures to factory workers.

The national health institute was the nucleus of health policies in Czechoslovakia; while the 13th district served as a social laboratory where the model of healthcare organisation and social intervention – campaigns and public education – could be tested. Hynek Pelc, a Rockefeller Foundation grantee, senior lecturer in social hygiene at the Charles University (Prague), was an active member of the institute in support of Procházka's project. He participated in many activities organised by the League of Nations. The scheme was supported by the Ministry of Health and Physical Training, and the Rockefeller Foundation gave financial support for the first five years. A series of social and medical organisations became members of the institute: dispensaries for children; Care for Youth; the Masaryk League against Tuberculosis; Czechoslovak Red Cross; Protection of Mothers and Children; Association against Venereal Diseases; and the Fire Brigade (with its Samaritans).

The first Czechoslovak rehabilitation centre for alcoholics was established in a consulting room for mental hygiene in 1928. It dealt with other addictions and mental problems and was managed by a psychiatrist. The board included a social committee, a committee of local district and consultancy doctors, the district health-insurance company, the Prague Medical Office, as well as members of the local council. Procházka kept the power to supervise the functioning of the whole organisation. Hynek Pelc was the representative of the national health institute and became its director in 1938. Pelc was a respected member of the international network of public health experts and he prepared an analysis of the health demographics and future needs.

Procházka wanted to implement his plan by giving responsibility to district doctors for certain sectors of Prague. He was convinced of the necessary coordination of social work and health intervention. Procházka proposed that all authority would be in the hands of the senior and district doctors, who would be in contact with the local health administration – as well as other authorities. The medical team would also supervise preventive healthcare in the district. The senior doctor would control the health office, district doctors, and all staff in the healthcare centres and dispensaries. The local district centre of social and health associations would be responsible for managing the budget, and the distribution of the funds among all the institutions (which mostly came from municipal and state funds).[66]

From the very beginning, Pelc insisted on the importance of public health education. He established a study programme for health service personnel of all ranks that was integrated in the educational activities of the state health institute. Several departments of the institute were involved in the training activities for future employees of the public health administration.

The 13th district of Prague was intended to become the 'social laboratory' for the state health institute, and a tool for the reorganisation and decentralisation of the health service for the chief medical office in Prague. The results were less positive than expectations. Several years later, Procházka commented: 'The time was favourable for grand projects, but antipathetic as regard achievements.'[67] Pelc also admitted, in 1937, that the educational activity of the state health institute was unsuccessful. Moreover, the war and the difficult post-war years later worsened the situation.

Nevertheless, the early years of the '13th Model District' could be considered successful. In 1927 it was composed of public health staff and voluntary organisations. The nursing service was reorganised on a regional basis. Educational campaigns and public health interventions were started, as well as a project to build a site for all the organisations working on public health in the district. In addition, healthcare centres for children were unified and day nurseries were opened in a couple of districts, and a centre for the rehabilitation of alcoholics was also established. There were antenatal dispensaries for pregnant women and several campaigns against infectious diseases – focussed on diphtheria – were implemented with large-scale immunisations. One of the most important novelties was the role of the so-called social-health nursing sister, who assumed similar duties to visiting nurses in other European countries.

Although the plans initially were proposed for a period of five years, from the early 1930s the difficult international situation and great depression meant that references to the 'model district' disappeared. Despite an enthusiastic start, the local centres of social and health associations of the 13th district of Prague and the planned social and healthcare centres later suffered Nazi interference in the 1940s, and the association was formally ended in early 1950s.

Medical education on public health and social medicine was carried out by the state health institute. Some medical authorities criticised the institute because it was supported by the Rockefeller Foundation and inspired in transnational models – for this reason the Rockefeller Foundation may have gradually lost patience with the Czech approach.[68] In sum, the state health institute did not develop entirely as Pelc had intended. It had not become the centre of postgraduate education of public health experts for the Czech public administration. Nevertheless, many modern concepts of public health and bio-policies did take root. Sometimes those public health initiatives were seen as experiments, rather than stable programmes of social and political action. The principle was kept in mind by the post-war healthcare reformers, as well as the established network of social and healthcare institutions in Prague that had survived the war. The system of a district-based allocation of nurses, instead of a division according to medical specialisation, as established in the 13th district, was an important advance that was continued in subsequent reforms in Czechoslovakia.

The aspiration of the state health institute to become an educational counterpart of medical faculties in the field of social hygiene was not as successful as elsewhere in Europe. Medical faculties and associations resisted. The state health institute encouraged a discourse aimed at the basic problems of public health and medicine, in which the social approach was dominant. The integrative principle of the debates became prevention. Health centres, as defined by the European Conference on Rural Hygiene in Budapest and Geneva in 1931,[69] were similar to the pattern of the Czechoslovak 'national health institutions'.

The exemplary 13th district was called to implement the methods of social hygiene presented by the state health institute, but the aspirations of the institute and the school of hygiene were not finally realised. Only in the early years of its existence did it operate in accordance with its purposes. This was especially true as a teaching arrangement for the education of medical personnel, health and social nursing sisters, and as a source of statistical research. The work of the voluntary organisations and health officers was successfully coordinated. But ambitious plans to reorganise the Prague health office and to extend the system to other districts, faltered and eventually failed.[70]

Alfonso XIII National Institute of Hygiene in Madrid

In 1871 Spain established an *Instituto Nacional de la Vacuna* whose main task was to organise an anti-smallpox vaccination programme along the lines of similar institutions in other European countries. The centre was reformed in 1894 and changed its name to *Instituto Nacional de Bacteriología y de Higiene*, and this name was, in turn, replaced in 1900 by the *Instituto Nacional de Sueroterapia, Vacunación y Bacteriología Alfonso XIII*. The institute became the central national health institution covering areas of epidemiology, bacteriology, serum therapy, vaccination, parasitology, disinfection and veterinary medicine. In 1910 its name was again changed to the *Instituto Nacional de Higiene Alfonso XIII* (INHA),[71] and finally, when a republic was proclaimed in 1931, it became *Instituto Nacional de Salud* [National Health Institute].

A central health administration was established in Spain at the start of the twentieth century. A technical body called the *Dirección General de Sanidad* [General Health Directorate] was constituted in 1922.[72] A director-general of public health reported to the minister and coordinated the work of the technical and administrative officials working in three main departments:

1   The Inspectorate-general of the Interior, including the provincial inspectors of health and the provincial sanitary brigades. The Inspector-general of Health led 52 provincial inspectors in charge of the health situation in the province under their jurisdiction, especially with regard to deficiencies and measures to be taken in the case of infectious diseases. Efforts were made to improve notifications of preventable diseases and ensure that the municipal courts delivered suitable certificates in all cases of death from infectious disease. These officials received the daily death register for each district and coordinated actions with district and municipal inspectors in case of epidemics.

The provincial sanitary brigades (1921) carried out campaigns against infectious and parasitic diseases by deploying preventive vaccination, disinfection, and the early diagnosis of preventable diseases. It was also their duty educate the public in matters of hygiene using pamphlets, speeches, and movies. The brigades treated water and transported patients; some produced vaccines and sera, and undertook chemical and bacteriological tests of water and foodstuffs.[73] A central sanitary brigade coordinated the work.

2   The Inspectorate-General of the Exterior had to prevent infectious diseases and plagues, namely cholera, plague, and yellow fever, from entering in ports and crossing frontiers. District sanitary stations existed in the main coastal cities, islands, and colonies. These stations took care of disinfection and ran laboratories for diagnosis, accommodation for patients, and treatment of infectious diseases.[74] At the port sanitary stations there was also an antivenereal service.

3   The Inspectorate-General of Public Health Institutions was created in 1919. It had a national scope and was composed of:

   a)   Alfonso XIII National Institute of Hygiene (Madrid)
   b)   Royal Hospital for Infectious Diseases (Madrid)
   c)   Central Sanitary Brigade (Madrid)
   d)   Lago Anti-Tuberculosis Sanatorium (Galicia)
   e)   Sea Sanatoria in Oza, Pedrosa (Cantabria) and Malvarrosa (Valencia)
   f)   Health Statistics Service (Madrid).

It also dealt with sanatoria and leper colonies[75] and coordinated pharmaceutical and veterinary services. Attached to it were organisations and associations, dealing with health improvement, campaigns against venereal diseases, protection of mother and children, malaria, and tuberculosis. The administration was advised by the Royal Health Council, Royal Academy of Medicine, and provincial and municipal advisory bodies.[76]

The *Instituto Nacional de Higiene Alfonso XIII* assumed a wide range of activities: anthropometric and racial records, surveys of the health of the population, as well as preventive and hygienic measures and mapping disease territories.[77] Philanthropic associations were expected to contribute financial and human support to the foundation of the national institute, since bacteriological science enabled medical laboratories to produce sera and vaccines for the prevention of infectious diseases, such as diphtheria, rabies, tetanus, parasitic diseases, puerperal fever, tuberculosis and cholera. Spanish authorities recognised a delay in this field, and appealed to patriotism to reinforce the biopolitical arguments. The country was still reeling from the effects of the catastrophic Spanish-American War in 1898, and its leaders were very aware of the need to transform and modernise Spanish society. Moreover, national laboratories represented icons of modernity and scientific progress, as well as being a source of state revenue. Spain paid large sums to obtain products from the *Institut Pasteur*, which showed the wide benefits of medical-technical laboratories for cattle raising, biotechnologies, ferments, manures, and pest control, as well as enabling huge improvements in human health.

The new INHA was established in Madrid and organised into four fields of activities. The first area was devoted to general research on human biology. The second focussed on vaccination – initially, the anti-smallpox lymph. The third area concentrated on bacteriology, and analytic tests as requested by individuals and public authorities, as well as carrying out research on practical hygiene and micrography. The fourth area was devoted to serum therapy and produced and distributed anti-rabies vaccine, tuberculine, malleine, anti-diphtheria, anti-tetanus and anti-streptococcus sera, as well as all types of vaccines for avoidable epizootics – including anthrax, contagious pneumonia and cowpox. These four sections were assisted by chemistry and veterinary departments. In addition, there were kennels and stables for animals.

The institute carried out 4,371 vaccinations in 1923, produced a quantity of lymph sufficient for 1,092,147 vaccinations for state campaigns, and delivered 15,270 doses of anti-plague vaccine; 2,700 tubes of anti-plague serum; 27,000 doses of anti-typhus vaccine; 448 tubes of anti-diphtheria serum; 2,050 doses of anti-influenza vaccine; and 500 doses of anti-dysentery vaccine. Some 2,000 people requested anti-rabies vaccinations and 1,300 received a vaccination. The institute also performed 74 bacteriological and 44 chemical water tests and organised advanced courses in public health studies with 22 students.[78]

In addition to its work in practical preventive medicine, the Alfonso XIII Institute was actively engaged in scientific research. The institute's director for its first two decades was Santiago Ramón y Cajal, a neurohistologist awarded the Nobel Prize in 1906 for establishing neuron theory. As an expression of its research orientation the institute began to publish a quarterly *Boletín del Instituto de Sueroterapia, Vacunación y Bacteriología de Alfonso XIII* in 1905. The journal had a strong bacteriological focus and a dual aim of communicating the institute's research activities and summarising the latest international developments in bacteriology and public health. In addition, it contained an abstract section for foreign scientific publications and the work done in major European laboratories. The *Boletín* was edited by a group of researchers who concentrated on the bacteriological analysis of infectious diseases and serum-therapy. The INHA's activities thus followed the European pattern of national health institutes, as shown by a 1906 report on vaccination in several Western countries commissioned by the *Académie de Medicine* in Paris.[79]

After the First World War, the orientation of the institute changed. The publication of the *Boletín* was interrupted by financial problems and changes in the institute's scientific personnel and research orientation in 1919. Ramón y Cajal resigned the directorship in 1920. New staff were engaged and a hard redefinition of tasks and priorities took place. In 1922 a bulletin entitled *Archivos del Instituto Nacional de Higiene de Alfonso XIII* marked the start of a new age. Editor-in-chief was Francisco Tello, a pupil of Cajal, and the editorial board was composed of young researchers who were mostly linked to the League of Nations and the Rockefeller Foundation. In keeping with the scientific orientation of its editors, experimental research on infectious diseases dominated the pages of the new journal.[80] Indeed, the institute's new journal eliminated its predecessor's practice of reporting on international developments, assuming that the publications of the Pasteur Institute, the *Office International d'Hygiène Publique,* and others, were easily available to researchers. *Archivos* became an expression of the research activities conducted by the members of the Alfonso XIII Institute.

During the following years, the research undertaken at the institute paid special attention to malaria, a prevalent problem in several Spanish regions, although much research also focused on venereal diseases, laboratory technologies, serological reactions, leptospirosis, and Malta fever. Jorge Ramón and Fañanás recorded the statistics of anti-rabies campaigns; and research by the institute's parasitological department – led by Gustavo Pittaluga – was published by his pupils Emilio Luengo, Sadí de Buen, and P. Aznar under the title of *Trabajos de la Sección de Parasitología. Notas parasitológicas.*

The African colonies were a key focus for INHA activities before World War One.[81] The campaigns of preventive medicine coordinated by the institute concentrated on the most disadvantaged social groups suffering the worst living conditions and the lowest health standards. The poorest rural areas in the Spanish countryside and Spain's African colonies were obvious regions of interest, since they contained many whose poverty and health conditions posed a clear threat to national social hygiene. One of the institute's first large projects using clinical and experimental methods to improve public health was the Pittaluga expedition to explore sleeping sickness (*trypanosomiase*) in the Spanish colonies in the Gulf of Guinea.

Subsequent research commissions from the Alfonso XIII Institute dealt with other health problems in the colonies. In 1914 Francisco Tello, head of the epidemiological section, and his assistant Antonio Ruiz Falcó, published a report on the outbreak of plague in Casablanca in 1909 which had affected several districts of Morocco. The report included excellent ethnographic documentation about the living conditions of the population. It contained a chronicle of the activities, an epidemiological report, clinical observations, bacteriological analyses, a medical topography of the affected area, and an assessment of future risks for the district.[82] At the same time, a change in the orientation of colonial health policies was proposed to include recognition of and cooperation with the indigenous authorities in order to improve efficiency. The work of the Pittaluga commission in Guinea was cited as an example of the importance of access to indigenous bodies.

Combatting malaria in rural Spain became the chief goal with the aid of the Rockefeller Foundation. Dealing with domestic health issues remained the core responsibility of a national institute of health. Therefore, the third example of the institute's engagement dealt with in this chapter is the anti-malaria campaign in rural Spain. The initiative began in 1920 as an experimental project led by a committee chaired by Gustavo Pittaluga and funded by the Rockefeller Foundation. A research station was established in a district of the Cáceres province which was severely infested with malaria. Here techniques and procedures were tested that were subsequently used in the national campaign. This started at the end of 1921 and followed a pattern of clinical examination, blood testing, pharmacological treatment, permanent supervision, inspection of homes and water supplies, improving the sanitary conditions of the soil, treatments with pesticide, epidemiological research and technical training. The institute's national campaign against malaria was based on an intensive and multi-factorial programme of diagnostic and therapeutic medical intervention.[83] The anti-malaria campaign was much more ambitious than the previous campaigns against colonial diseases.[84] It involved a larger group of public health experts from both national and international institutions and required more complex laboratory support.[85]

The campaign also entailed increasing the number of rural doctors and health assistants in malarial districts and upgrading their skills in the field. Sadí de Buen, Gustavo Pittaluga, and Emilio Luengo, all of them public health experts and members of the Alfonso XIII Institute, organised a course to instruct 11 rural doctors that included a practical campaign in the province of Cáceres. In Navalmoral, the city council refurbished a municipal building to act as a centre in the fight against malaria: it included large areas for teaching and research, and small rooms for patients.[86] Further courses to instruct doctors in the anti-malaria fight were organised in 1926 in collaboration with a network of rural health centres in Cáceres (Dr Morote), Córdoba (Dr Benzo), Badajoz (Dr Bardají), as well as 35 days of practical training for students at the *Escuela Nacional de Sanidad* and coordinated by Sadí de Buen. Rural doctors appointed for a job in anti-malaria services could also take a course at the *Escuela Nacional de Sanidad* (National School of Hygiene, Madrid) followed by a practical assignment in Navalmoral. The anti-malaria campaign in Spain aimed at eradicating the disease and extending local medical expertise in experimental laboratory technologies.

These instructional activities yielded good results thanks to the financial support of the Rockefeller Foundation, which helped to increase field staff and improve working facilities, including the organisation of a specialised library. This collaboration also made a mobile service possible that was based on laboratory tools and facilities for clinical screening and examination in specialised tents similar to those used in military campaigns. It worked on the Jerte riverside and in the fight against anopheles using a chemical called *Paris Green.* The latter were of great interest for practical training in the use of this new larvicide. Funds from the Rockefeller Foundation enabled a group of doctors to work with the provincial anti-malaria service, and a doctor who worked on a long-term basis in Navalmoral was also paid to assist the Las Hurdes Royal Board.[87]

The Spanish project received international recognition and public support. Between 13 August and 7 September 1925, the King of Spain, the Director-General for Health, the Inspector of Health Institutions, the Inspector of *Sanidad Interior*, and the League of Nations' Committee for Malaria all visited Extremadura and reviewed the organisation of the anti-malaria campaign. The League of Nations Health Committee sent two doctors for practical experience with the anti-malaria programme in 1926 and 12 in 1927. The health department's technical commission described the campaign's work in two detailed reports published in 1926.[88] All these events confirm the medico-political importance of the project and the international interest it received. Charles Bailey, a delegate of the Rockefeller Foundation, visited the laboratories and technical facilities and supervised programmes from the very beginning, returning several times accompanied by Alfred Russell, Director of the International Health Board of the Rockefeller Foundation, and W. Strode, Head of the Rockefeller Foundation for Europe. Foreign medical researchers, such as Roël, Aldo Castellani, M. Langeron and F.O. Gaillard, visited rural areas as well. Poor rural Extremadura became a field for international anti-malaria intervention, as described by Sadí de Buen in 1928:

> Thanks to Dr Bailey's proposals, we could send several of our technicians abroad. Dr Luengo spent nine months in the United States studying at the *School of Hygiene and Public Health* at the *Johns Hopkins University* and working in the field; doctors Sánchez, Peralbo (1926), Ortega and Oquiñena (1927) attended a course organised by the League of Nations in Paris under the direction of Dr Brumpt, and they then travelled for two months in several malaria districts, the latter two accompanied by doctors Martín Cano and Torrademé, with board and lodging paid by the League of Nations; I myself [Sadí de Buen] spent five months in the United States and one month in Italy.[89]

The campaign to eradicate malaria was the most important health programme in Spain from a technological viewpoint. In 1925–1927 services and dispensaries were operational in 13 provinces: Madrid, Toledo, Cáceres, Badajoz, Huelva,

Córdoba, Seville, Avila, Salamanca, Murcia, Alicante, Tarragona and Barcelona. They were equipped for the fight against mosquitos and mosquito larvae and offered patient screening, pharmacological treatment, and soil quality improvement. The Malaria Commission, a technical board named by the central committee, assisted those centres with instruments, facilities, and free quinine. Most of the municipal and provincial health services were connected with the activities of the Malaria Commission, which also surveyed endemic malaria in many other rural areas of Spain. An increasing number of provincial health inspectors launched municipal and provincial anti-malaria services, following the commission's guidelines.

Health propaganda and education for the general public were an important part of the commission's activities. Houses with some kind of mechanical protection against mosquitoes were distinguished with an award; posters and leaflets were distributed at schools; technical publications were circulated, and a film was produced by the Rockefeller Foundation to record the practical activities of students of the National School of Health during their stay at Navalmoral. Lectures and courses were delivered in rural districts in several provinces. Scientific material from the malaria campaign was also used for instructing specialists at the medical faculties, in the training courses of the INHA, and wherever requested by Spanish or foreign entities.

A significant volume of research generated by the campaign was published in international journals. A new type of *Spanish recurrent fever* was described by Sadí de Buen within the framework of his malaria research,[90] and studies were also conducted on transmission paths, biology of anopheles, geographical distribution of the disease, and effectiveness of pharmacologic treatment (principally based on quinine, alkaloids and plasmoquine). The geographical distribution of kala-azar was also surveyed. Gil Collado, an entomologist, collaborated with the Commission and the country's top specialists in health statistics. Marcelino Pascua did fieldwork in Navalmoral for several months to create a permanent system of epidemiological records. The commission tried to appoint an engineer specialising in malaria in 1927, but the proposal was not accepted for financial reasons.

A report on the campaign against malaria (1925–1927), published in 1928, included a detailed description of the work done in each district. Dispensaries and hospitals coordinated resources for treatments, with research and teaching being the main activities. Dispensaries contained an office to receive patients, a room for clinical screening, and a laboratory for blood analysis. Each patient had a chart containing identity details, age, clinical records, clinical screening – with special reference to the spleen – parasitological blood analysis and other data. Drugs for malaria, recurrent fever, Malta fever and kala-azar were distributed free of charge. The malaria dispensary was managed by local doctors assisted by nurses. The Navalmoral hospital had five rooms: three small rooms for children containing seven beds, one for men with four beds and another one of the same size for women. Malaria patients were not commonly hospitalised but, over two years, 142 patients were admitted to hospital due to tertiary and quaternary fever, laverania, esplenomegaly, kala-azar, recurrent fever, Malta fever, and ancylosto-miasis. Treating these hospital patients enabled researchers to study the effects of drug therapy in malaria, kala-azar and recurrent fever.

Preventative clinical trials were also developed with assistance from the Rockefeller Foundation. In the trials, preventive quinine was given to control groups and curative quinine to patients with an infection. Eliseo de Buen coordinated these field services together with three assistants. They received two Ford cars and all the necessary materials from the Rockefeller Foundation, which also funded a modern laboratory and a specialised library. Malaria stations developed techniques to catch mosquitoes and larvae, which were studied and artificially bred at the laboratory. Stations also had some meteorological equipment. Statistical records, and epidemiological maps, were compiled by Marcelino Pascua.

During the period of republican government (1931–1939) and a few years before the civil war (July 1936), the name of the INHA was changed to the *Instituto Nacional de Salud* [National Health Institute]. It was conceived under a reformist government programme that was handicapped by budget reductions. Nevertheless, there was a consensus about the need for a new institution to coordinate and improve sanitary research and public health policies. The prevalent ideology considered that scientific research and improving the teaching of sanitary staff would become the main milestone for sanitary reforms and deepen the scientific policies developed by the National Board for Scientific Research and the Rockefeller Foundation collaborative programmes.

Shortly before the new National Institute of Hygiene was created in 1934, a paper by G. Pittaluga, S. de Buen, and M. Benzo discussed at the First National Conference of Health [*Congreso Nacional de Sanidad*] (Madrid, 1934) analysed health policy and proposed a coordinating institution to manage scientific research. The aim was not 'high level scientific research', but for research programmes focused on an applied strategy to solve the main health problems. It was argued that a central institution could organise research lines and strategies and better publicise research results.

Just a few months later, Pittaluga took charge of the new institute. However, the objectives were not fully accomplished as fragmentation persisted in practical terms as the same staff and facilities remained in place. The state-led reformist programme in social medicine was abandoned in 1936 as a consequence of the civil war. The situation worsened after the war due to a lack of material and human resources mostly associated with political reprisals applied by Franco's regime and the exile of numerous scientists and doctors.[91] A health act was published in 1944 and then developed by regulations in 1946. Public health and preventive medicine were not priorities in medical care and hospital assistance. Technology took centre-stage. The Spanish health system during Franco's regime followed completely different patterns to the European liberal democracies and the result cannot be considered a state welfare project. Medicine lost, in many senses, its political dimension as a tool for social health.[92]

Public health institutes in Scandinavia

Statens Serum Institut in Denmark

The *Statens Serum Institut* was inaugurated on 9 September 1902 in Copenhagen to produce and supply anti-diphtheria serum to the population. Its first director was Carl Julius Salomonsen.[93] At the turn of the century, diphtheria was a severe infectious disease and treatment by serum from horses previously vaccinated by the toxin reduced mortality rates by half for patients suffering from the disease. As a transnational phenomenon, the establishment of the institute coincided with the international expansion of national health institutes promoting preventive medicine based on experimental microbiology and immunology.

Shortly after its establishment, SSI undertook a series of new assignments consisting of the development of several sera, vaccines, bacteriological and serological diagnostic tests, and the production of epidemiological records, as well as cooperation in the fight against epidemics. During the interwar years, the fight against tuberculosis was given a high priority in Denmark and other Scandinavian countries. Tuberculosis patients were registered and rates were surveyed, special dispensaries were established to take care of patients. Chosen by the Health Organisation of the League of Nations as a reference laboratory for testing biological and serological products, SSI headed the development of tuberculin for diagnostics and the development of the tuberculosis vaccine BCG, which already in the 1930s was used for the vaccination of people exposed to tuberculosis in regions such as Greenland. In the 1920s, the SSI was the leading enterprise for developing pertussis vaccine; and in the 1930s the Danish Institute took over the production of the pertussis vaccine, participated in the develop-ment of the first Danish foot-and-mouth disease vaccine, and developed vaccines against tetanus and diphtheria.

This very active and ambitious programme of research and social medicine was led by prominent experts such as Thorvald Madsen and established the Copenhagen Institute as an international benchmark for the standardisation of sera and vaccines. Madsen was the president of the Health Committee of the League of Nations between 1921 and 1937 and later became one of the active founders of the World Health Organisation. Together with the leaders of the Rockefeller Foundation International Health Division and Ludwik Rajchman, Witold Chozko, Léon Bernard and Andrija Stampar, he was one of the most influential figures in international health during the interwar years.[94] As direc-tor of the State Serum Institute, Thorvald Madsen conducted the first scientific investigations into the use of pertussis vaccine as a treatment during an outbreak on the Faroe Islands in the North Atlantic in 1923–1924. Vaccination using whole bacteria inactivated by phenol or formalin mitigated disease morbidity and mortality when compared to unvaccinated controls. Another epidemic in 1929 yielded additional promising results.

Tuberculosis and typhoid epidemics led to the establishment – with the support of the Rockefeller Foundation – of an epidemiological department at SSI. The main objective was to survey the incidence of infectious diseases and participate in their prevention and treatment. In the 1920s, SSI produced the first blood-type serologic reagents and performed blood-typing serological tests for Danish hospitals. In 1932, the voluntary blood corps of the Boy Scout and Girl Guide Associations and Voluntary Boys' Brigade were attached to the SSI, and SSI then undertook supplying blood and blood products to Danish hospitals. For a number of years SSI led one of Denmark's largest blood banks.

The International Salmonella Centre started work in 1938 under the management of Fritz Kauffmann. The centre worked for international standardisation and typing of the more than 2,000 known types of salmonella. Kauffmann also developed sera for treating severe pneumococcal infections.

After World War Two, the Serum Institute was active in the international tuberculosis conferences and campaigns. It was managed by the Dr Johannes Holm in Copenhagen. Fifty-seven million children and young people, mostly in Central Europe, were tested for tuberculosis with tuberculin produced by SSI, and 16 million were vaccinated against tuberculosis, mostly receiving SSI's BCG vaccine. The volume of these sera and vaccines shows the importance of the Danish Institute. Furthermore, this first mass international vaccination became a role model for World Health Organisation's vaccination campaigns, especially in connection with strategies for the eradication of smallpox. International cooperation was always very important to the SSI. The Institute participated in international networks and trained scholars from developing countries in laboratory techniques and vaccine production.

The Norwegian Institute of Public Health

During the initial decades of the nineteenth century, following independence in 1814, the Norwegian government activities in public health were mainly limited to smallpox vaccination campaigns, expanding medical training, and increasing the number of district medical officers.[95] Sixty-three officers were active in 1836, while the number had doubled by 1854. However, as elsewhere in Europe, the incursion of cholera provoked a comprehensive rebuilding of the framework of public health organisations and campaigns. In May 1860, a royal commission published a public health act regulating public health boards and actions to control epidemics and contagious diseases. It established the fundamentals of primary healthcare, preventive medicine, municipal public-health administration and central state institutions. Each commune established a health board, composed of representatives from local government and the community, which was presided over by a district medical officer, as the representative of the central health authority. Proposals from municipal health boards were submitted to the communal council prior to approval from the central government. However, the activities of health boards were constrained by limited economic resources and, in some cases, by the political ideology of communal councils.

Legislation in 1860 established the framework for initiating public-health policies in Norwegian communes. However, the central health authority was weak, lacked resources, and its primary activity was compiling and publishing national health statistics based on annual reports produced by the district medical officers. Consequently, public health measures varied a great deal throughout the country. In large towns, health services became highly developed, and employed new technologies such as X-rays, whereas in many rural communes, health boards were inefficient.[96]

From the late 1880s, professional associations, charitable societies, and political parties increasingly advocated public-health campaigns. The Norwegian Medical Association was established in 1886 with the aim of promoting public health policies. Professional organisations for midwives and nurses pushed in the same direction. The expansion of public health and the spread of a hygienist mentality, together with a labour movement that demanded the public right to healthcare, prompted new legislation regarding conditions at schools, regulation of foster children, food quality control, hygienic working conditions and housing, and similar issues. Local health boards and district medical officers played an advisory and supervisory role. The establishment of the national women's charity, *Norske Kvinners Sanitetsforening* (NKS) [Norwegian Women's Public Health Association] in 1897 gave rise to a large public health movement in Norwegian society that mobilised considerable sums of money and thousands of volunteers.[97] The NKS supported many projects such as the establishment of childcare clinics and nursing homes, although its central activity was focused on the fight against tuberculosis.

The national campaigns against tuberculosis began in 1900, when new national legislation increased the capacity of public-health authorities to act for the protection of society. Tuberculosis had become the most frequent cause of death in Norway, especially widespread among the most productive sector of society: young adults.[98] District medical officers were to register and monitor all patients suffering from the disease. They could determine specific measures such as disinfection and compel hospitalisation by using, if necessary, the police.[99] In the following years a network of mostly publicly-owned sanatoria and hostels was built. At its climax, it included over one hundred institutions managing over three thousand beds. Public hospitals and health centres cared for the patients, while the *Norske Kvinners Sanitetsforening*, together with other charity associations and the National Association Against Tuberculosis (1910), used large public information campaigns to prevent the transmission of the disease. Legislative compulsion was extended to include mandatory chest x-ray screening from 1942 and mandatory tuberculin testing and BCG vaccination from 1949. Tuberculosis appeared as a terrible threat in Norway, similar to syphilis in most European countries.

In 1912 the Norwegian parliament approved a reorganisation and substantial expansion of healthcare services. The number of primary medical officers in municipal and rural districts was increased from 161 to 372 and a new office for the county medical officer was created to act as an intermediate link between districts and the central directorate of medical affairs under the Ministry of Social Affairs.[100] Three years earlier mandatory sickness insurance for about one-third of workers had been enacted. This legislation expressed public engagement in healthcare matters including the construction of hospitals, public baths, a school medical service, dispensaries for pregnant women, infants and young children.

During the economic crisis, new questions appeared relating to food and nutrition. In this field, the famous 'Oslo breakfast' received international acknowledgement and became a strategic reference for several European countries. But a series of *biopolitical* issues associated with the expansion of social medicine came under discussion: especially regarding social hygiene, sexuality, and racial hygiene. Throughout most of the interwar period, however, economic depression weakened public finances and therefore many programmes were abandoned.

The Norwegian Institute of Public Health (NIPH) was founded in 1929.[101] Initially, the institute was responsible for providing vaccines and sera, and performing chemical analyses of water and food. Some years later, the NIPH implemented immunisation programmes, but for several decades the scope of the institute was restricted to infectious disease control. The institute's name changed from *Statens Institutt for Folkehelse* [State Institute for Public Health] to *Nasjonalt Folkehelseinstitutt* [National Institute of Public Health]. Its new role as national coordinator in several fields emphasised the importance of cooperating with universities, hospitals, and other research institutes – and a series of national collaborating groups were formed.

The NIPH had 18 employees in 1929 and its budget was extremely small, amounting to just NOK 107,000. Most of the employees were volunteers. Clean water and safe food were perhaps the most important factors for a healthy population, and one would therefore presume that the idea of a state laboratory was met with praise. Surprisingly, pharmacists strongly opposed the idea, probably because they feared that a state laboratory would take over their responsibility for performing chemical analyses. It took another 40 years before parliament, after a heated debate, established a state laboratory. The Board of Health Laboratory in 1916 was established at the premises of the State Hospital of Norway.

The Board of Health Laboratory became a pillar in the construction of a national public health institute. Another pillar was the Animal Vaccine Institute founded in 1891, initiated and headed by the doctor and veterinarian Ole Malm (1854–1917). The institute's only task was to produce smallpox vaccine, smallpox being one of the two most feared infectious diseases at the time, together with tuberculosis. Whereas there was no pharmaceutical treatment for tuberculosis, smallpox could be effectively prevented through vaccination and, therefore, producing the necessary vaccine was of the utmost importance.

The Norwegian Institute of Public Health was based on a donation from the Rockefeller Foundation. The decision to establish a national public health institute was made in 1916 when parliament passed the proposal to found a Board of Health Laboratory, but the name Institute of Public Health was not used before the new building had been inaugurated in 1929. The Board of Health Laboratory merged with the Animal Vaccine Institute, and three other small laboratories and units, to form a new and larger institution. It was not merely the name that changed – the Norwegian Institute of Public Health was a completely new institution and similar to the others we have previously discussed. It was also supported by the Rockefeller Foundation. Eighteen staff moved into an impressively large and modern laboratory building in 1929. The stables were soon filled with horses and sheep, and the animals turned into production units for various types of therapeutic sera. Initially, the institute had five departments: bacteriology; chemistry; syphilis serology; a department for provision of vaccines and therapeutic sera; and a department for animal vaccine production.[102]

By 1935 the institute was producing therapeutic sera against diphtheria, bacterial meningitis, tetanus, streptococcal disease, and typhoid fever; and vaccines against gonorrhoea, typhoid, paratyphoid infections, staphylococcal and streptococcal infections, as well as smallpox. In addition, human polio serum was imported from France. As infectious diseases were the most important threat, control became the main task of the institute. Drinking water control was another important duty, and during the war a department of blood typing and immunology was also established.

A re-evaluation and renewal of state public-health initiatives began with the Labour Party's election in 1935, but efforts were suspended by war and occupation. The start of the construction of the Norwegian welfare state after 1945 caused a reorientation of public health policy under the leadership of Karl Evang. In his vision, public health was an integral part of the welfare state. Achievement of this goal required the expansion of preventive healthcare, which would be carried out by *distriktsleger* [district medical officers] assisted by specially trained *helsesøstre* [public health nurses] and supervised by *fylkesleger* [county medical officers]. It also required the rationalisation of the country's many small local hospitals into a network of large central hospitals with specialist institutions for chronically ill patients.

Notes

1   Baldwin, P. *Contagion and the State in Europe 1830–1930*, Cambridge: Cambridge University Press, 1999.
2   Canguilhem, G. *Le normal et le pathologique*, Paris: PUF, 1966; Foucault, M. *Il faut défendre la société*, Paris: Éditions du Seuil, 1997.
3   Latour, B. *The Pasteurization of France*, Cambridge, MA: Harvard University Press, 1988.
4   Latour, B. *Reassembling the social: An introduction to actor-network-theory*, Oxford: Oxford University Press, 2005.
5   Ibidem, p. 5.
6   Ibidem, pp. 5–6.
7   Labisch, A. *Homo Hygienicus. Gesundheit und Medizin in der Neuzeit*, Frankfurt am Main: Campus, 1992.
8   Latour, *Reassembling the social* (2005), p. 39.
9   Ibidem.
10 Ibidem, p. 123.
11 Debré, P. *Louis Pasteur*, Baltimore: Johns Hopkins University Press, 1998; Geison, G.L. *The Private Science of Louis Pasteur*, Princeton: Princeton University Press, 1995; Carnino, G. 'Louis Pasteur: Pure science serving industry', *Mouvement Sociale*, 248, 2014, pp. 9–28.
12 Carnino 'Louis Pasteur: Pure science serving industry' (2014), pp. 9–12; Debré, *Louis Pasteur* (1998), chapter 1; Geison *The Private Science* (1995).

13 Hulverscheidt, M.; Laukötter, A. (eds) *Infektion und Institution. Zur Wissenschaftgeschichte des Robert Koch-Institus im Nazionalsozialismus*, Göttingen: Wallstein Verlag, 2009; Brock, ThD. *Robert Koch. A life in medicine and bacteriology*, Berlin: Springer Verlag, 1988; Gradmann, Ch. *Krankheit im Labor: Robert Koch und die medizinische Bakteriologie*, Göttingen: Wallstein, 2005; Schultz, MG. 'Robert Koch', *Emerging Infectious Diseases*, 17 (3), 2011, pp. 548–549.

14 Hüntelmann, A.C. 'Staatliche und kommunale Gesundheitspflege vor und nach dem Ersten Weltkrieg', in Hofmann, W. (ed.) *Fürsorge in Brandenburg: Entwicklungen, Kontinuitäten, Umbrüche*, Berlin: Be.Bra Wissenschaft Verlag, 2007.

15 Hulverscheidt; Laukötter (eds) *Infektion und Institution* (2009).

16 Ibidem.

17 Schultz, 'Robert Koch' (2011), p. 548.

18 Wilkinson, L.; Hardy, A. *Prevention and cure: the London School of Hygiene & Tropical Medicine: a 20th century quest for global public health*, London: Kegan Paul Limited, 2001.

19 Cook, G.C. *From the Greenwich Hulks to Old St. Pancras. A History of Tropical Disease in London*, London: Bloomsbury Academic Collections, 2015.

20 Johnson, R. 'Colonial Mission and Imperial Tropical Medicine: Livingston College, London, 1893–1914.' *Social History of Medicine*, 23 (3), 2010, pp. 549–566.

21 Cook, *From the Greenwich Hulks* (2015).

22 Johnson, 'Colonial Mission' (2010), pp. 551–553.

23 Barona, *The Rockefeller Foundation* (2015).

24 Ibidem.

25 'Letter from the Secretary-General of the League of Nations to the Foreign Office, 18th February, 1924 regarding the Establishment in London of a School of Hygiene'. LONA, 1213/34087, 1924.

26 Barona, *The Rockefeller Foundation* (2015).

27 Wilkinson; Hardy, *Prevention and cure* (2001), p. 3.

28 Cook, *From the Greenwich Hulks* (2015), p. XII.

29 Cook, *From the Greenwich Hulks* (2015), p. 5.

30 'Memorandum on the Organization and functions of the Ministry of Health (England and Wales)'. Ministry of Health, March 1925, Geneva: LONA, 123/47764/26249, 1925.

31 Ibidem.

32 Johan, B. 'The Training of the Public Health Officers in Hungary'. Geneva: LONA, C.H.630, 1927.

33 'Letter from Selskar M. Gunn to Norman White on sanitary reforms in Hungary'. Geneva : LONA, 1283/29308/26249, November 19, 1925.

34 Bélan Joan was an active member in the training commission of the League of Nations, participating as well in the conferences of national schools of hygiene.

35 Andreja Stampar was the Croatian leader of public health initiatives in Yugoslavia during the interwar years.

36 This was the normal way of action of the RF: funding initiatives they had previously agreed with national authorities.

37 Balinska, M.A. 'The National Institute of Hygiene and Public Health in Poland 1918–1939'. *Social History of Medicine*, 9, 1996, pp. 427–445.

38 Balinska, 'The National Institute' (1996), pp. 82–83.

39 Ibidem, pp. 83–84.

40 Barona, *The Rockefeller Foundation* (2015), pp. 59–65.

41 Balinska, 'The National Institute' (1996), p. 431.

42 Barona, *The Rockefeller Foundation* (2015), pp. 59–65.

43 Barona, *The Rockefeller Foundation* (2015), pp. 59–65; Rose, W. 'Epidemic control in Europe, and the League.' *American Review of Reviews*, 46, 1922, p. 2.

44 'Institute of Hygiene [in Poland]', Terrytown, New York : RAC, IHB Minutes, 5th May 1922 and 23rd May 1922, RG 1.1. series 789, box 1, folder 1.

45 Balinska, 'The National Institute' (1996), p. 433. Letter from W. Rose to Rajchman, 6 July 1922. Archives of the Joint Distribution Committee, New York, File 362.

46 Balinska, 'The National Institute' (1996), p. 433.

47 Balinska, 'The National Institute' (1996), p. 434.

48 Ibidem.

49 Ibidem.

50 Balinska, 'The National Institute' (1996), p. 435.

51 Balinska, 'The National Institute' (1996), p. 442.

52 'Décret Ministériel sur l'établissement et organisation de l'Institut Central d'Hygiène à Belgrade', Geneva: LONA, 1924.

53 Dugac, Z. 'Like Yeast in Fermentation: Public Health in Interwar Yugoslavia.' In: Promitzer, Ch.; Trubeta, S.; Turda, M. *Health, Hygiene and Eugenics in Southeastern Europe to 1945*, Budapest: Central University Press, 2011, p. 195.

54 Dugac, 'Like Yeast in Fermentation' (2011), p. 207.

55 Ibidem, p. 208.

56 Másová, H. 'Social hygiene and Social Medicine in Interwar Czechoslovakia with the 13th District of the City of Prague as Its Laboratory', *Hygiea Internationalis. An Interdisciplinary Journal for the History of Public Health*, 6 (2), 2007, pp. 53–68.

57 Másová, 'Social Hygiene and Social Medicine' (2007), pp. 54–55.

58 Ibidem.

59 Ibidem, p. 55.

60 Ibidem, p. 56.

61 Ibidem, p. 60.

62 Ibidem, p. 60.

63 Ibidem, pp. 60–62.

64 'The State Hygienic Institute, Prague, Czechoslovakia. Outline of the working program of the Institute', Geneva: LON Archives, 1925.

65 'The State Hygienic Institute' (1925).

66 Másová, 'Social Hygiene and Social Medicine' (2007), p. 65.

67 Ibidem.

68 Ibidem.

69 Barona Vilar, J.L.; Cherry, S. (eds) *Health and Medicine in Rural Europe (1850–1945)*, Valencia: Publicaciones de la Universidad de Valencia/Seminari d'Estudis sobre la Ciència, 2005.

70 Másová, 'Social Hygiene and Social Medicine' (2007), pp. 66–68.

71 On the complex antecedents of the institute, see Porras Gallo, M.I. 'Antecedentes y creación del Instituto de Sueroterapia, Vacunación y Bacteriología Alfonso XIII', *Dynamis*, 18, 1998, pp. 81–106.

72 Porras Gallo, 'Antecedentes y creación' (1998), p. 368.

73 Ibidem, pp. 368–369.

74 Ibidem, p. 369.

75 All legal sources are joined in Navarro García, R. *Historia de las Instituciones Sanitarias Nacionales*, Madrid: Instituto de Salud Carlos III, 2001.

76 Barona, *The Rockefeller Foundation* (2015).

77 For the role of technology creating racial and national identities, see Medina, R. 'Extracting the Spanish Nation from Equatorial Guinea. Scientific Technologies of National Identity as Colonial Legacies'. *Social Studies of Science*, 39, 2009, pp. 81–112.

78 *Bulletin de l'Office International d'Hygiène Publique*, 1923.

79 Serret, R. 'La vacuna en el extranjero'. *Boletín del Instituto de Sueroterapia, Vacunación y Bacteriología de Alfonso XIII*, 2, 1906, pp. 177–182.

80 Buen, Sadí de; Luengo, E. 'Poder tripanolítico del suero de un enfermo tratado por el Bayer 205', *Archivos del Instituto Nacional de Higiene de Alfonso XIII*, 2, 1923, pp. 53–56; Buen, Sadí de; Luengo, E. 'Ensayos terapéuticos con el "Bayer 205" en dos casos de tripanosomiasis humana', *Archivos del Instituto Nacional de Higiene*

de Alfonso XIII, 2, 1923, pp. 85–96; Luengo, E. 'Nuevas investigaciones en un caso mortal de tripanosomiasis humana tratado por el Bayer 205'. *Archivos del Instituto Nacional de Higiene de Alfonso XIII*, 3, 1924, pp. 203–210.

81 Barona Vilar, J.L. 'In the Name of Health. The *Instituto Nacional de Higiene Alfonso XIII* and laboratory campaigns in Spanish rural áreas and African colonies, 1910–1924'. In: Andresen, A.; Gronlie, T.; Hubbard, W.; Ryymin, T. (eds) *Health Care Systems and Medical Institutions*, Oslo, Novus Press, 2009, pp. 154–169.

82 Tello, F.; Ruiz Falcó, A. 'La peste bubónica en la zona de influencia española en Marruecos'. *Boletín del Instituto de Sueroterapia, Vacunación y Bacteriología de Alfonso XIII*, 10, 1914, pp. 97–143.

83 Rodríguez Ocaña, E. *et al.*, *La acción médico-social contra el paludismo en la España metropolitana y colonial del siglo XX*, Madrid: Consejo Superior de Investigaciones Científicas, 2003.

84 Comisión Central de Trabajos Antipalúdicos. *Memoria de la campaña contra el paludismo (1925–1927)*, Madrid: Ministerio de la Gobernación, Dirección General de Sanidad, 1928.

85 Barona, 'In the Name of Health' (2009), pp. 159–164.

86 Comisión Central (1928), p. 5.

87 Comisión Central (1928), p. 6.

88 Swellengrebel, N.H. *Informe sobre el viaje a España.* Boletín Técnico de la Dirección General de Sanidad. Marzo, 1926. Madrid: Comité de Paludismo, Ministerio de la Gobernación, Dirección General de Sanidad, 1927.

89 Comisión Central (1928), p. 7.

90 Buen, Sadí de, 'Note préliminaire sur l'épidemiologie de la fièvre recurrente espagnole', *Annales de Parasitologie humaine et comparée*, IV, 1926, pp. 185–192.

91 Barona, Vilar J.L. (ed.) *El exilio científico republicano*, Valencia, PUV, 2010.

92 On the history of the post-war successor to the Alfonso XIII Institute, see Nájera Morrondo, R. 'El Instituto de Salud Carlos III y la sanidad española. Origen de la medicina de laboratorio, de los institutos de salud pública y de la investigación sanitaria', *Revista Española de Salud Pública*, 80, 2006, pp. 585–604.

93 Salomonsen, C.J. (ed.) *Contributions from the University Laboratory for Medical Bacteriology, to celebrate the inauguration of the State Serum Institute*, Copenhagen, O.C. Olsen & Co., 1902.

94 Borowy, I. *Coming to Terms with World Health. The League of Nations Health Organisation 1921–1946*, Frankfurt am Main: Peter Lang, 2009.

95 Hubbard, W.H. 'Essay Review. Public Health in Norway 1603–2003'. *Medical History*, 50, 2006, pp. 113–117.

96 Ibidem.

97 Ibidem.

98 Ryymin, T. 'Tuberculosis-threatened Children: the Rise and Fall of a Medical Concept in Norway, c. 1900–1960'. *Medical History*, 52, 2008, pp. 347–364.

99 Hubbard, 'Essay Review. Public Health in Norway' (2006), p. 115.

100 Ibidem, p. 117.

101 *History of the Norwegian Institute of Public Health.* https://www.fhi.no/en/about/about-niph/this-is-the-norwegian-institute-of-public-health/history-of-the-norwegian-institute-/ [Accessed 10th July, 2017].

102 Elvbakken, K.T.; Ludvigsen, K. 'Medical Professional Practices, University Disciplines and the State: a case study from Norwegian Hygiene and Psychiatry 1800–1940', *Hygiea Internationalis*, 12 (2), 2016, pp. 7–28.

6 Instructing the experts
National schools of public health

Teaching the experts: more than a national issue

Previous pages have shown to what extent national schools of public health played a crucial role in the creation of an international network of experts in public health and social medicine policies. Expert networks were extremely influential over national policies. Indeed, national schools had a national scope, but were in fact shaped, discussed, coordinated, and promoted by influential international players. Should the schools be part of the university system or independent institutions integrated in the state health administration? The answer to this question depended on national academic traditions, political organisations, and the struggle between professional interests and public administration. At the inauguration of the Budapest and Zagreb Schools of Public Health (1927) a conference was held for the directors of the national schools in several European countries, with the participation of several members of the Health Committee of the League of Nations. In his report on the training of public health experts at this meeting, the French hygienist and political authority Léon Bernard stated:[1]

> In brief, one truth emerged from this debate – that it would be a mistake to advocate a rigid system. The relations between Schools of Public Health and Universities and public health administrations must vary according to circumstances; there are only three essential principles, embodied in the absolute rule that the existence of such relations is indispensable. The first principle is that the staff and services both of the University and of the health administration must cooperate with the School of Public Health. Second is that the Governing Bodies of Schools of Public Health should include representatives both of the Universities and of the health administration, whatever may be the formal system of establishment and management or the size and development of the schools, this being dependent upon the stage reached in the education of public opinion on the subject of public health. The third principle is that the schools should be permeated by a scientific spirit and yet at the same time preoccupied with its practical applications; any school which disdained the scientific ideal would lower its standard and gradually decline, and, once cut off from the true source of all educational life, it would soon be

discredited and die. In the same way, if a professor in such a school lost the taste and capacity for applying his knowledge and his teaching in practice, his own faith would soon wither.

The enunciation of these principles demonstrates both the complexity and the high intellectual level of the controversies carried on at the Conference; and it should be of service for the guidance of bodies and individuals concerned with the organisation of Schools of Public Health.

This text of Léon Bernard summarises most of the controversial issues and open questions at the time. National schools for the teaching of public health experts were expanded throughout most European countries during the 1920s. This event is perhaps in part a consequence of a spirit of emulation, as well as a necessary requirement in the process of professionalisation. Schools were mostly supported by national authorities, in many cases with the direct intervention and financial support of the Rockefeller Foundation. Should the schools be a part of the university organisation or part of the central state administration? Should they essentially care for practical problems or do experimental research as well? These topics will be discussed in the following pages. Four meetings of directors of European national schools took place in the late 1920s, the first in Budapest, and subsequently in Zagreb, between 29 September and 4 October 1927. The agenda addressed four principal issues: comparing national programmes; attracting and selecting students; the relations between schools of public health, universities, and the public administration; and the cooperative relations between public health schools in different countries.[2]

Comparative programmes of public health schools

During the 1927 conference, H. Pelc, the director of the School of Public Health in Prague, prepared a report summarising the programmes of the different schools in European countries and specialist university courses on hygiene.[3] After this global perspective, several participants summarised the situation in their respective countries. The Pole W. Chodzko contributed very valuable information and made a lucid analysis of the programme introduced in Warsaw.[4] The Croat Andrija Stampar then explained the successful health programme in Zagreb.

> Consideration of these reports and the discussion which followed led to the conclusion that no system of uniform programmes for all schools could be contemplated. Many and various factors enter into the question: the position and stage of development of the school itself, the material, technical and social conditions under which it has to pursue its aims, the stage of progress reached by the national health institutions for which it has to provide, the standard of education previously attained by its students, and lastly the customs and ethnography of the peoples among whom the experts trained at the school will be called upon to work.[5]

There was a general agreement that the programmes of all schools should be based on certain general principles, and while the broad framework should be uniform in view of their purposes – the methods, number, duration, and standard subjects taught must vary according to local conditions. The agreed reference was always the wide scope and high standard of the School of Public Health at Johns Hopkins University, led by William H. Welch. Welch studied at Yale University (1870) and did his medical training at Columbia University (1875), served as an intern at Bellevue Hospital, and widened his expertise at a series of European universities – including Strasbourg, Leipzig, Breslau, and Berlin from 1876 to 1878. After his return to Bellevue Hospital Medical College, Welch was appointed professor of pathological anatomy and general pathology. When he joined the hospital and school of medicine at Johns Hopkins (1884), he had a huge international experience and wide perspective. He held posts at the School of Hygiene and Public Health, as well as the Hospital and the School of Medicine. He served as dean of the medical faculty and was the first director of the School of Hygiene and Public Health and the Institute of the History of Medicine, and one of the founders of the *Journal of Experimental Medicine* (1896). He served as president of the board of directors of the Rockefeller Institute for Medical Research (1901–1932), being advisor to John D. Rockefeller, for the funding of the Peking Union Medical College. His extensive experience matched his capacity to influence.

Attracting students for schools of public health

When dealing with the audience of the national schools of public health, W. Chodzko summarised four targeted groups: medical officers; general practice doctors; private practitioners; and social workers.[6] As regards the instruction of health officers, in certain countries like the UK, the government required that the officers hold the diploma of a specialist school, considered to be the only sound system for the public health instruction. It was assumed that the efficiency of experts trained in specialist schools was guaranteed. The British regretted that this rule had not been adopted in every European country and argued that governments should only employ reliable and competent professionals. Therefore, administrations should regulate specialist training and require an official diploma. Chodzko emphasised the great importance of instituting specialist courses in preventive medicine for general practice doctors. He quoted George Newman's statistics: in one part of England out of 107.795 general patients treated in 1924, 76% were suffering from preventable diseases. The 3,048,397 patients treated in 1925 by 159 insurance funds in Poland, Chodzko found that 63% of the cases could be regarded as preventable.[7] It would therefore be desirable in the interest of public health, economy, and finances, that general practice doctors be trained in the precepts and practice of preventive medicine.[8] At Warsaw an agreement was signed with local sickness insurance funds with more than 400,000 members, municipal health services, and the state railways, for the organisation of a course on preventive medicine for their doctors.[9]

Relations between schools of public health, universities, and public health administration

The American, W.H. Welch opened the discussion on the development of the essential concepts of public health and distinguished three stages – each having a different objective as its essential characteristic: firstly, sanitation; then the prevention of disease; and finally, active social hygiene. The extension of the field of public health led to the need for specialist schools able to embrace the whole of this large, complex, and varied series of subjects. Welch defended that these schools should confine their work to the application of the general principles of the scientific spirit, but independently of universities and the public health administration – although in close collaboration. Others, including the Croat, A. Stampar, considered that the health administration, being responsible for public health, should establish schools of hygiene to train their own officials, as in Yugoslavian institutes of public health, whose work was linked to the universities in terms of lectures, facilities, teaching activities, and public education programmes.

Schools of public health could be officially incorporated into the university system, or even as a part of the medical faculty. However, certain points of criticism were discussed: some argued different orientations existed because medical faculties were mainly focused on curative medicine, while public health schools dealt with preventive medicine. Nevertheless, for many diseases (such as diphtheria, malaria, tuberculosis, or syphilis) treatment involved not only prevention, but also therapeutic and social hygiene. A change in the orientation of medical faculties by devoting more attention to preventive action was necessary, so that medical practitioners could cooperate with the officials acting in public health services.

The same argument served to answer the second objection: that the teaching of public health in medical faculties was almost negligible. The argument was that the preventive perspective should be essential in courses on public health, and in all courses and teaching posts. As the teaching of public health and preventive medicine required specialist equipment that was only available at specialist schools, there was no reason why such a school should not be part of a university. In this way, the specialist schools could benefit from the influence of university organisation and make available to medical students the use of the apparatus conceived and installed on a large scale for the use of specialists in public health.

Cooperation between schools of public health

A very central issue regarding the efficiency of schools of public health, received the most valuable suggestions from Bélan Johan,[10] director of the Budapest School and W. Chodzko.[11] Both contributions were carefully discussed by the conference. The final agreement assessed the positive interaction that periodical meetings of directors of schools of public health contributed. Interchanges of staff members from different schools were considered very productive, especially when including assistants and technical staff, rather than professors or senior researchers. Schools were also called to exchange publications, and endeavour to include in their publications summaries, in major languages, of the papers published. The directors also considered the possibility of publishing joint reports explaining the work, organisation, and activities of each school. Nevertheless, the most important resolution of the Budapest and Zagreb meetings concerned joint research into questions of immediate and common interest. Those issues show the common viewpoints and collaborative attitude among the leaders beyond political and scientific conflicts. Those leaders constituted international elites governing public health policies in the European national administrations.

National schools and public health experts

National health authorities shared a nuclear idea: they believed that the training of public health experts was the cornerstone to implementing health policies nationally and internationally. This was also the viewpoint of the leaders of the League of Nations Health Committee and Health Organization, shared by the Rockefeller Foundation International Health Board. In January 1923, the Health Committee decided to survey the programmes of specialisation in public health and preventive medicine at European, Japanese, and American universities. On 20 February 1924, the League of Nations created a Permanent Commission on Education in Hygiene and Preventive Medicine consisting of eight international health specialists, including the Spaniard Gustavo Pittaluga. The Commission was presided by the French hygienist and LNHO leader, Léon Bernard. The dean of the medical school in Shanghai joined the commission in 1930.

The international initiatives taken by those institutions included coordinating and institutionalising. One initiative was to collect and publish information on how healthcare services were organised and how they operated in the several European countries (national sanitary regulations, identification of health problems, and private institutions involved). This was a task traditionally done by the *Office Internationale d'Hygiène Publique* since its establishment in 1907. A second initiative was to promote a network of leaders, interchanges, and interactions between countries by funding visits of public health experts to study and discuss healthcare systems and policies.[12]

The organisation of travelling exchanges involving health experts in different countries was an initiative developed by the Secretariat of the League of Nations and the health authorities in different countries. The International Health Board of the Rockefeller Foundation supported the programme and generously funded exchange visits – the first of them taking place in October 1922. Some visits were available for public health officers; others involved specialists in tuberculosis, children's health, school hygiene, health administration, health control of ports, epidemiologists, and so on. After eight years at work, by 1930 some 600 officers had taken part in the exchange visits of sanitary staff. These visits included countries that were not members of the League of Nations, such as the United States of America, Mexico and the Soviet Union. Among the visited nations were most European countries, the Latin American nations, Canada, Western African nations and territories, India, and Japan.[13]

In some cases, the Rockefeller International Health Board/Division took over state responsibility in sanitary matters. In Spain, for example, public health experts sponsored by the RF ensured the implementation of new technologies. The two international organisations were closely associated. Basically, the LNHO depended on funds provided by the RF: between a third and a half of its budget came from American philanthropy, and RF experts intervened directly in the proposal, planning, and development of League health programmes. Between 1922 and 1927, the RF contributed $350,000 to institutionalise the LNHO's statistics programme and epidemiological studies. Between 1922 and 1929 it provided $500,000 to promote the exchange of public health experts. Some authors state that during 1930–1934, the RF donated $2,700,000 to fund a library and a centre of documentation in public health at the LNHO offices in Geneva, although the project was never fully implemented.[14]

The Health Committee of the League also allocated individual grants to instruct public health experts and health officers abroad, and assist them in diffusing new techniques and organisational strategies for the expansion of health administrations in their respective countries. The programme of study grants was designed by the LNHO after assessing the sanitary and social conditions of the home country of the candidates. The League established a teaching commission in 1925, and in 1927 it conducted two international courses on hygiene in London and Paris to improve specialist qualifications. We shall offer some details on these courses in the last part of this chapter. Experts from around 20 countries attended these courses.

Interwar Spain provides a good example of the public health training programmes supported by the RF and the League. Official contact between the RF and the Spanish government was established in the early 1920s. In 1924 a delegate of the Rockefeller Foundation, Charles Bailey, started a series of reports on the public health situation in Spain.[15] He paid special attention to the recently created *Escuela Nacional de Sanidad* [National School of Health], describing its organisation, functioning, teaching staff, and training programmes. He predicted a difficult future for the school because it lacked experts who could carry out practical instruction in laboratory techniques. Experts and technology were the institution's weak points according to Bailey. Furthermore, teaching staff were poorly paid and devoted only a part of their time to official duties. They often had several jobs, and sometimes owned private laboratories. To improve the level of expertise of Spanish public health personnel, a programme of study grants (mainly in the United States, but also in some European institutions) was approved, and over the following decade 23 young Spanish doctors were supported for at least one year of instruction in public health abroad.[16] These fellowship holders represented the vanguard of a new public health administration in Spain, and several were especially active planning an ambitious sanitary reform during the republican period (1931–1936) and the civil war (1936–1939).

Soon after its constitution, the League of Nations Permanent Commission on Education in Hygiene and Preventive Medicine decided to investigate three main topics in various countries in order to gain a comparative perspective: (1) training of experts, medical officers, engineers, architects, nurses and public health staff; (2) the extent of public health teaching for medical students and general practitioners; (3) public health instruction to teachers, priests, civil servants and others active in health education.

The commission designed a project to implement teaching public health in medical faculties, programmes for experts in schools of public health, a survey of the health condition of the population, materials for professionals, propaganda, public education programmes, and the teaching of hygiene in schools.

During the successive meetings of the commission, wide-ranging reports were produced on the situations in Austria, Finland, France, Germany, Hungary, Italy, the United States, and Yugoslavia. Reports were presented by Thomasz Janiszewski, Minister of Health in Poland (1922–23); Josephus Jitta, President of the Council on Health in the Netherlands; Bernhard Nocht in Germany; and Dr Timbal, Director General of the Public Health Service in Belgium. Public health teaching in France was reported by Léon Bernard, one of the founders of the Health Organisation of the League of Nations, while Donato Ottolenghi reported on some Italian cities, and George Newman, Chief Medical Officer to the UK Ministry of Health reported on the situation in Britain. Finally, Carl Prausnitz, expert member of the LNHO, described the situation in Germany.[17] This group represented the elite European leadership in public health and health administration.

The vast amount of information collected by the teaching commission led to a series of publications and international conferences focussed on the coordination of teaching strategies. Obviously, decisions were not imposed on individual states, but were negotiated in a context of the growing international influence of expert authority and a general spirit of internationalism. The first international conference bringing together the heads of national schools of health took place in Warsaw in 1926 just after the inauguration of the Polish National School of Health.[18] A second conference was held in Budapest and Zagreb in 1927 on the official opening of national schools in Hungary and Yugoslavia, while the two most important conferences took place in Paris and Dresden in 1930.[19]

During its meeting in Warsaw in 1926 the Commission of Public Health Instruction urged regular meetings between directors of national schools to exchange views on various problems, discuss the best method of promoting health instruction, and consider possible cooperation activities. The League Health Committee was invited by the Government of Hungary and of the Kingdom of the Serbs, Croats, and Slovenes to the opening of the schools of public health in Budapest and Zagreb (funded by the Rockefeller Foundation).[20] On the inauguration of the schools, a conference of directors took place in Budapest from 29 September until the 4 October. Two members of the International Health Division of the Rockefeller Foundation attended this meeting: W.L. Mitchell, member for Hungary, Rumania, and the Kingdom of the Serbs, Croats and Slovenes; and Dr Milam, member for Austria, Czechoslovakia and Poland.

After considering the reports and the remarks of the directors and the rest of the participants at the meeting, the conference reached a series of conclusions. There was a general agreement that standardising public health schools in different countries was not desirable. Programmes in each country depended on local conditions and requirements and, therefore, the orientation of programmes could vary according to local needs and traditions. A formula should be found for each country to establish the right proportion of theoretical instruction and laboratory work.

Once more, on the relations between public health schools, universities, and the health administration, opinion coincided that close cooperation should be combined with the need for autonomy, since universities and schools served different purposes, and should develop independently from each other. Close cooperation between universities and schools would be advantageous to help establish a proper balance between curative and preventive medicine. The difference between university institutes and schools regarding scientific and experimental work lay in the immediate practical importance of the health problems. At the same time, the participants at the conference highlighted the need for a very close relationship between the schools and public health services, and even the need for freedom from administrative interference. Public health schools aimed to become official technical organisations under the central health administration. In a previous conference held in Warsaw, William H. Welch, director of the Johns Hopkins School, showed the plurality of situations in each country and proposed three principles: collaboration between the three institutions; participation of university representatives and health authorities in the school management boards; and the combination of science and research with a practical engagement with the real demands of the population.

In terms of recruitment of students, apart from medical officers in the service of the administration, many non-medical personnel employed in the various branches of the health administration could be recruited: engineers, administrative officials and school teachers. Special attention was to be paid to arranging courses for insurance company doctors, owing to the growing importance of health insurance organisations in the prevention of diseases in many countries. But recruiting students from groups other than medical officers in the service of the state naturally depended on the existence of organised groups receiving instruction in public health and on legal provisions for courses at the school. It was recognised that this strategy was very important for propaganda and public education campaigns. A decisive factor in ensuring an adequate demand depended on the social prestige and salary of medical officers, compared with the earnings of practicing doctors.

Directors were anxious to establish links for close technical collaboration. The similarity between the health problems they had to challenge justified the view that cooperation would be valuable and that direct exchange of experiences was desirable. Representatives from Budapest, Prague, Warsaw, and Zagreb – as well as other institutes in the Kingdom of Serbs, Croats and Slovenes – met in a subcommittee and made a list of proposals:

1 Sharing results of research regarding treatment of scarlet fever. Exchange of antigens and sera and discussion regarding the most effective preparation and methods; properties of the preparations being tested by national commissions consisting of laboratory, clinical, and epidemiological experts; standardisation of the preparations by the final method agreed.

2 Mutual verification of tests for the serological diagnosis of syphilis with a view to the introduction of uniform methods. The uniform application of methods and testing techniques, as well as the periodical exchange by various institutes of the antigens employed and sera obtained from patients, and assessing when the disappearance of a positive Wassermann test in the serum varies according to the blood group of the patient.

3 Evaluation of the effectiveness of oral vaccination against typhoid fever using the Besredka method. Using comparative methods in districts with widespread endemic foci and in institutions with a resident population: prisons, orphanages, asylums and so forth. They proposed that all residents and inmates be vaccinated as far as possible.

4 Joint study of the methods of water analysis and measures for the control of water supplies, with a view to selecting measures and standards most suitable for the conditions of the countries concerned. The sub-committee considered that the standards used in the United States and Great Britain had not proved to be applicable to all countries.[21]

5 Commitment to solve the most urgent problems of hygiene: water supplies, drainage, purification of drinking water, especially in rural districts. It was therefore proposed 'to hold a competition between the institutes for the construction of a model latrine and a model well and for the best method for the purification of drinking water in wells and small containers'.[22]

6 Reciprocity for licensing of certain therapeutic preparations.

7 Exchange of information, reprints, and documents, in three languages: English, German, and French.

The Conference decided to request the assistance of the Health Organization of the League of Nations in carrying out these proposals, in particular, coordinating comparative studies regarding prevention and treatment of scarlet fever, expansion of the Wasserman test, and oral vaccination techniques. The League could also advise the national schools and institutes concerning the other questions raised, especially for reciprocity for licensed preparations, appointment of a jury for the latrine competition, arrangements for an exchange of technical staff for a closer contact between institutions, and arrangements for further director conferences.

A third international meeting of directors of public health schools took place in Paris in 1930. The main topic was the international homologation of teaching programmes, as well as the professional profile of the experts taught at the national schools of public health.[23] The specific topics addressed were the number of departments, specialist areas, teaching programmes, practical training, associated scientific research, length of the teaching period and practical training, diplomas, and the role of health schools in policies and administration. Various reports from the London School of Hygiene and Tropical Medicine[24] were presented by Andrew Balfour. Other papers referred to the State Institute of Public Health in Prague by Bohumil Vacek and Hynek Pelc,[25] the functioning of the Social Work School in Prague and the School of Public Health in Warsaw by Marcin Kacprzak.[26] A general open discussion about experiences in the national schools of health in each country was stimulated, and aspects such as the role of health officers, teaching organisation, practical training, scientific research, and health engineering were also in the agenda. Andrija Stampar, head of the Zagreb School and prominent participant in the network of experts, contributed a paper on the organisation and activities at the schools of hygiene,[27] and the Hungarian Bélan Johan explained the training of health officers in his country.[28] Carl Prausnitz, professor of public health in Breslau, synthesised the general conclusions.[29]

Directors of European public health schools met in Dresden in July 1930 and focussed on the establishment of a minimum common programme of training for health officers and the teaching of preventive and social medicine to medical students.[30] A subcommittee devoted to analysing the role of public health museums in the public education on hygiene was established. The commission's activity promoted the professional profile of the public health experts and the fundamental role of health officers. National schools of public health schools defended their role in teaching experts and developing a collaborative networking strategy that included Baltimore, Zagreb, Budapest, London, Dresden, Prague, Warsaw, and Madrid. Between 1924 and 1930, the heads of public health schools held regular meetings and participated in an international debate about specialist training and its relation to public health policies. Although this activity was formally sponsored by the LNHO, the RF emphatically supported it by giving technical aid, grants, project funds, and providing an integrative international framework.

In his final report to the Paris conference (1930), Carl Prausnitz focused on the central role of the medical health officer, but he also referred to the general practitioner, sanitary staff, and the general population, especially teachers and scholars. Prevention and public health should become the new ideology, and social mobilisation involving trade unions and religious institutions was needed. Prausnitz's report insisted on the fundamental difference between expert knowledge and popularisation in terms of language, materials, and orientation.

The concluding report approved by all participants underscored several points. It was agreed that schools of public health were essential for health policies and teaching experts – and should function as technical institutions independent from the general public administration, political power, and universities. It was also agreed that several institutions exhibited the desired profile: in the United States these included the Johns Hopkins School of Public Health, the Harvard school, and several others, mainly funded by the Rockefeller Foundation; while in Europe, these included the national schools established in Madrid (1924, reformed in 1930), Warsaw (1925), Budapest and Zagreb (1926), London (1929), Prague (1930), and Athens (1930).

The American model was based on universities and the European model mostly on state institutions. France and Germany followed different patterns, but cooperation with university staff was considered essential. The aim of these institutions was to teach public health administration experts and educate the public about hygiene. They should link research and teaching, offer practical training, as well in laboratory technologies, and lead sanitary campaigns. Research was an essential expression of the so-called *scientific spirit*, but it should not be conducted independently from the practical problems of the population. In certain European regions, previous experience showed the positive effects of practical action for specific programmes.[31]

The fifth point on the agenda was the agreement on a common curriculum for the training of medical officers at national schools. The proposal consisted of a comprehensive course of study ranging from specifically medical subjects, taught in lectures and the laboratory, to instruction in the social, political, and administrative aspects of public health.[32] The minimum approved curriculum was:

a)   General hygiene, including lectures and practical laboratory training in physiology, physics, chemistry, bacteriology, immunology, serology, parasitology, entomology.

b)   Clinical training in diagnosis and treatment of acute infectious diseases.

c)   Sanitation as applied to housing in urban and rural communities.

d)   Vital statistics and epidemiology including lectures and practical training.

e)   Elements of sociology, especially regarding the environmental and social conditions influencing health and disease, eugenics, and physical education.

f)   Social services and dispensaries for prenuptial couples, pre-birth maternities, infant and child care, social and school hygiene, tuberculosis, venereal diseases, cancer, alcoholism, mental and physical deficiencies, poverty, and local problems such as malaria, trachoma, leprosy, lice, and so on.

g)   Industrial hygiene.

h)   Hospitals and other healthcare services.

i)   Social insurance.

j)   Public education campaigns.

Moreover, practical training in rural areas for at least three months was recommended as an essential part of the instruction to become a public health officer. Students should play an active role in all fields: organising social hygiene programmes, sanitation, public health administration, and health campaigns. States were urged to demand that candidates for posts in public health services, whether national or municipal, be graduates of a national school of health. This practice had produced excellent results in several countries, and was recommended as a rule. As we will see, the professional profile of public health experts was submitted to a transnational negotiation and the international network put pressure on governments.

The Dresden conference further proposed that schools adopt a pattern of management based on a director or a dean supported by an administrative board with several departments organising teaching and research activities led by full-time professors and at least two part-time assistants. Professional stability and full-time dedication were central points, with external specialists contracted only for specific topics.

In sum, those meetings tended to influence the establishment of a common profile of professionalisation for public health experts, and created an internationally agreed scheme for national schools of public health. This was a powerful tool to spread a hegemonic pattern of knowledge and expertise, and legitimate political action and social intervention. Health officers and inspectors were the key element for training medical practitioners, public health assistants, and other complementary staff, as well as organising public campaigns. Public health schools should adapt their facilities to the newest laboratory technologies, give lectures, implement public education campaigns, and gather teaching materials in hygiene museums for educating children and the general public.

Promoted by the Rockefeller Foundation and the LNHO Health Committee, the schools flourished during the interwar years as crucial institutions to legitimate international public health expertise and *biopolitical* intervention. International conferences of directors of public health schools framed the international debate about specialisation and public health expertise – and so shaped a common pattern of organisation, instruction and action. Statistics and experts, together with state policies, became essential elements for social medicine.

The international model: Johns Hopkins School of Public Health in Baltimore

The Johns Hopkins School of Public Health was opened in the autumn of 1918.[33] It was initially supported by an annual grant of $250,000 from the Rockefeller Foundation. In February 1922, the RF increased this annual fund to $5,000,000 and made a further appropriation of $1,000,000 for the construction of a suitable building for facilities, laboratories, and offices. For seven years, the school occupied temporary quarters in the former laboratories of the university. Plans for the new building had been made in the spring of 1922, but construction was delayed and it was not finished until 1925.

The school was organised not as a department of medicine, but as a separate school with an independent faculty, coordinated with the other university faculties. In 1926, it consisted of 13 full professors, seven associate professors, nine associate researchers, three instructors, 12 assistants, and five extramural lecturers. Faculty belonged to nine different departments: public health administration; epidemiology; biometry and vital statistics; medical zoology; bacteriology; immunology; physiological hygiene; chemical hygiene; and filterable viruses. One or more trimestral courses were arranged in each of these scientific fields, including laboratory and seminar work. In addition, opportunities were offered for advanced work and research. Separate lectures were given on specialist topics, such as mental hygiene, quarantine, and sanitary regulations. Finally, provision was made for fieldwork with health departments during the summer months.

Two principal purposes guided the establishment of the school. Firstly, to provide suitable professional training to medical graduates entering public health. Secondly, to support and develop research work in the field of hygiene and public health. The various scientific fields represented in the departmental division were prominent emerging research areas, which eventually became fruitful areas of development. The Johns Hopkins School became the world reference centre for public health instruction.

Two higher degrees were granted. One was a Doctor of Public Health, open to graduates in medicine, awarded after the satisfactory completion of six trimesters of work at the school and at least one trimester of fieldwork with an official public health agency. In general, four of the six trimesters were given to lectures, while two trimesters were devoted to advanced work in one department, including the preparation of a thesis.

The other degree was Doctor of Science in Hygiene. This was offered to graduates in arts and science, as well as to graduates in medicine, with certain specialist requirements regarding previous training. No set curriculum was arranged for candidates for this diploma. The work done was almost wholly in one subject, and included the satisfactory completion of a research project. Usually, three years of graduate work was required, but the actual time necessary varied with the previous training. A certificate in public health was awarded to graduates in medicine who had satisfactorily completed three trimesters of work in certain subjects. In addition to candidates for degrees and certificates, the school received many American and foreign students who came to study in one or more departments and who remained for varying periods of time (taking courses or engaging in advanced work).

The building was located adjacent to both Johns Hopkins Medical School and Johns Hopkins Hospital and occupied part of the medical centre. It housed all the facilities except sanitary engineering, which was taught in the engineering laboratories of the university. The organisation and activities of the several departments are summarised below.

Department of Public Health Administration

The department shared space with the Department of Epidemiology on the second floor of the building. The activities involved did not require complex equipment and a general lecture room was the most often used room. The Office of Administrative Information of the US Public Health Service worked on collecting surveys and materials on administrative procedures from American health departments and on the classification and analysis of statistical records. These materials were made available for teaching and research in the school. A space was assigned to the local Office of Shellfish Sanitation of the Public Health Service, and so making available to members of staff and students the materials used in that area of public health work. The department had a work room equipped with a calculator, an office for the secretary, a room for preparation of mimeographed materials used for teaching, a small seminar room, as well as work room for specialist students, and a store room.

Teaching was based on field demonstrations and conferences. An introductory lecture course of two hours a week during the first trimester was given for orientating students beginning the subject, particularly those from overseas, in the historical development and fundamental principles of American health administration. During the second trimester a course of four hours a week was devoted to the study of the administrative problems involved in public health. Research was focused on the health administration in the United States. Statistical surveys of administrative information from the Public Health Service formed the basis of most research.

Department of Epidemiology

As epidemiology is too comprehensive to be taught in a single department, instruction focused on epidemiological problems that face administrative health officers in their work. With few exceptions, students entering courses in epidemiology were medical graduates with a knowledge of pathology. They usually had supplementary training in bacteriology and were required to have completed at least an elementary course in statistics. The Department of Public Health Administration introduced them to the rationale and organisation of administrative control measures. Consequently, students acquired a fairly broad knowledge of epidemiology and some command of clinical, bacteriological, and statistical techniques.

Instruction in the Department of Epidemiology was focussed on the methods of collecting field records of infectious diseases for comparing and supplementing experimental approaches. As it was impossible for the School of Hygiene to maintain the staff needed for entirely autonomous investigations in the field, and a primary requisite was a working connection with administrative public health organisations. Such connections existed with the city and state health departments, with the US Public Health Service, and other agencies. The head of the department was an officer at the US Public Health Service on active duty in the Division of Scientific Research.[34] The staff in 1926 consisted of a professor, an associate professor, an associate researcher, a secretary, and two technical assistants.[35]

Certain fields of research required the support of a laboratory for bacteriological and immunological diagnosis, but the need was filled by collaboration with the departments of immunology and bacteriology, and there was no need to set up a separate laboratory for epidemiology. A small car was used for fieldwork.

The course consisted of lectures and laboratory work (given throughout the second trimester) during three mornings a week. Lectures were devoted chiefly to the discussion of a series of field surveys selected to illustrate methods of research and the principles of reasoning applied to the interpretation of evidence. Lectures started discussing several sharply localised mass-infection epidemics of typhoid fever and other frequent diseases, describing investigations in progress, and analysing the rather complex processes of reasoning by which conclusions were reached. The discussion of more complex studies regarding the distribution of epidemic infections followed, as well as patterns for the interpretation of results, factors concerned in the prevalence and efficacy of control measures in specific instances, and so on.[36]

Laboratory work consisted of a series of clearly defined problems, similar to those previously discussed in lectures, which each student was expected to work individually. In general, the material given consisted of the following:

1 A set of research collected data.
2 A statement of facts essential for the interpretation of the statistical material.
3 Notes stating the problem and outlining the procedure to be followed for analysis.

Students tabulated the data to make an appropriate summary and presented the facts concerning the general epidemiology of the disease and their interpretation of the stated problems. Written analysis was returned to the teaching staff for review, marking, and subsequent discussion with the student. Work on each problem required an average of one or two weeks and the whole number of assignments in the course did not exceed eight or nine weeks. Instructors were always present in the laboratory for the necessary explanations and advice, but the policy followed was to let the student find his own way as far as he could.

A supplementary course in descriptive epidemiology was given as an elective choice in the afternoons during the second trimester – consisting of lectures given by lecturers on the epidemiology of the most common infectious diseases. Weekly clinics in the Municipal Hospital for Infectious Diseases, and research by each student of epidemiology on some disease not taken up in the lectures were also included. Students who wished to pursue studies in the department, beyond the established courses, were assigned to work on individual problems. The annual budget of the department was approximately $13,500; $11,500 for salaries and $2,000 for current expenses (the largest being transportation, maintenance of the small car, and occasional fieldwork).[37]

Department of Biometry and Statistics

The department of biometry and statistics was composed of a lecture room, general student laboratory, drafting and photographic rooms, and rooms for sorting, tabulating, and filing punched cards, as well as several offices for staff and graduate students, a laboratory, library, and storage rooms.[38] The department had a system of punched cards for analysing data, and research involving very large amounts of tabulation were handled in this way. The photographic section was well equipped for preparing charts and presentation slides. The supply of drawing instruments enabled the use of graphical methods of analysis for statistical issues. The department owned 43 computing and adding machines. One room was equipped as a probability laboratory containing a sampling machine used for experimentally testing the various types of sampling formulae. The department library stored data on statistics and contained about 4,000 statistical publications from cities and nations worldwide.

The department followed a specific programme of instruction. All candidates for the certificate and degree of doctor of public health course took an initial course in statistics three days a week during the fall trimester (consisting of lectures and laboratory work). Lectures dealt with statistics and statistical method, and these were amplified at the laboratory, where students under the guidance of instructors, were trained in the practical problems of collection, classification, and tabulation of statistical data, and in methods of statistical analysis. In the laboratory, students were given instruction in the use of punched cards, sorting, and tabulating machines. Students were also trained to use graphical methods – both for analysing material and presenting results.

Advanced courses in statistical method were offered for a more thorough knowledge of the analysis of experimental data, statistics, long time movements of population as a statistical mass, and population characteristics (such as birth rates, death rates, key indices, prevalence rates, etc). Three general headings summarise research lines: mathematical statistical method; analysis of existing statistical records in biology; and statistics.

Department of Medical Zoology

The department consisted of four divisions: protozoology; helminthology; medical entomology; and filterable viruses (although this was planned as a separate department). It contained a large lecture room used for courses in protozoology, helminthology, medical entomology, parasitology, and filterable viruses. A two-unit room was used for seminary meetings, and held the departmental and Samuel Taylor Darling Library. A series of small rooms contained a refrigerator, centrifuge, instruments, glassware, and chemicals, with technical assistants available to assist students and researchers. There were four rooms for small animals (guinea pigs and canaries) and larger animals were housed on the ninth floor.

Thirty-two students could be accommodated in the large laboratory, although classes usually ranged from 15 to 20 students, the courses mostly being electives, and chiefly taken by students who came from the tropics, or who expected to work in the tropics after completing their education. The staff consisted of three instructors in protozoology, three in helminthology, two in medical entomology, and two in filterable viruses. Other researchers and students did research as fellows – as part of the Rockefeller Foundation – research assistants and visiting researchers.

Research was published with other departments in the annual volume of collected papers of the School of Hygiene and Public Health. In the 1920s, the most important topics of research were bird malaria, trypanosome infections, intestinal flagellates, herpetomonads of insects and plants, hookworm disease, schistosomiasis, rat nematodes, intestinal flukes, anopheles mosquitoes, sand flies, measles, smallpox, and cancer. Various members of the department did fieldwork in Alabama, Trinidad, Puerto Rico, Honduras, Brazil, China, and Georgia.

The budget for work in medical zoology, exclusively for filterable viruses, was $25,635 of which $3,750 was for running expenses. Funds from outside sources almost equalled those from the school: approximately $25,000 during 1925–26 for the study of anopheles mosquitoes, hookworm disease and bird malaria.[39]

Department of Bacteriology

This department was focussed on teaching bacteriology to students of public health and for research in bacteriology. Lectures prepared students for the organisation and administration of public health laboratories in which the identification of the pathogenic organism was the most important aim.[40] Students were trained in systematic bacteriology to differentiate bacteria, also in sanitary bacteriology or bacteriological examination of air, water, soil, sewage, milk, and foods (to detect pathogens). The department offered two main courses in 'sanitary bacteriology' and 'public health bacteriology', and two specialist courses in 'food bacteriology' and 'spirochaetology' (the bacterial group called *spirochaetae* caused diseases such as syphilis, yaws, lyme disease, and relapsing fever).

Finally, there was a course for teachers in 'elementary bacteriology'. It was arranged for teachers who were active in teaching hygiene in public schools.[41] A seminar for the discussion of problems in bacteriology and immunology was organised in association with the department of immunology.

The research emphasis in 1926 was on the action of chemical disinfectants on bacteria in accordance with a fund provided by the firm Sharp and Dohme of Baltimore and New York. Candidates for the doctorate of science degree remained in the department for two to three years and most of their time was devoted to the investigation of a specific research problem in bacteriology, which served for their doctoral thesis. The majority of graduate students aimed to teach bacteriology or applied for public health laboratory positions. All candidates for doctor of science degrees who were taking their major work in bacteriology took the four main courses offered by the department.

A large teaching laboratory was provided with capacity for 40 students. A smaller laboratory for 15 students was provided for food bacteriology and courses on *spirochaetae*. There was also a small chemical lab, seminar, lecture rooms, and animal quarters. The department had a regular staff of seven: professor; associate professor; two associates; one instructor; one assistant; and one research assistant. The budget for 1925–26 was $23,000 ($15,000 for salaries, $5,000 for technical assistants, and $3,000 for current expenses).

Department of Immunology

The department was endowed with a laboratory for general class work, quarters for advanced students, private laboratories for members of staff, a preparation unit, and quarters for large numbers of laboratory animals. Its main functions were teaching and research. Teaching was offered in two ways: general class work for beginning students, and specialist work for advanced students. The course for beginners consisted of fixed exercises, for which the students were given detailed outlines and protocols covering the various kinds of serological reactions. They tested and standardised sera, while paying special attention to reactions that could be useful for diagnostic procedures. The theories and principles underlying these reactions were explained in lectures, conferences, and quizzes. The course was given twice a year. Moreover, a course for more advanced students was given in the spring trimester. The focus was on a small number of topics and no attempt was made to cover the whole subject of immunology. Scarlatine streptococcus, its toxin and antitoxin, was among the topics. Advanced students were given the opportunity to do research. The staff consisted of a professor, an associate professor, an associate researcher, a chief technician, a technician for the preparation unit, two assistant technicians, an animal caretaker and two assistants, and the annual budget $23,160 (with $4,796 for current expenses).[42]

Department of Physiological Hygiene

The practical work of public health agencies was largely concerned with the control of infectious diseases and protecting the public against the spread of epidemics. Moreover, another useful line of work was the study of how the body adjusts to the environment. From an individual perspective, experimental physiology dealt with the mechanisms for the maintenance of health and physiological hygiene. It also dealt with the physiological effects of change in the external environment, such as climatological change. A third subject was the study of industrial hazards in connection with sanitation and hygiene.

The department contained a large laboratory for class work, accommodating 50 students, equipped with work tables and outlets for gas, electricity, positive and negative pressure, and a dark room for photometric and visual experiments. The general lecture room accommodated 75 students and communicated with several smaller rooms for seminar activities. The air-conditioning plant was a complete installation designed to control the temperature, humidity, and movement of the air supplied to the lecture room and a specialist experimental room. Other rooms were used for special purposes such as refrigeration, centrifugal apparatus, weighing, distilling, sterilising, photographing, storing, and so on. Two rooms for X-ray and galvanometric work, contained a string galvanometer and the accessory apparatus to study muscular and nervous activity and fatigue. There were also animal rooms for small and large animals, equipped with suitable cages, floor drains, and a large steam sterilising apparatus.

The annual budget of the department was $24,150, and the staff included a professor, two associate professors, and two instructors, one for general physiology and other for industrial hazards.

Department of Chemical Hygiene

The department was equipped with a large student laboratory with space for 48 students with chemical tables endowed with appropriate apparatus (electric and vacuum drying ovens, electric centrifuges, and other instruments), while the wet wall was equipped with gas, water, electricity, vacuum and compressed air outlets. There were also service tables containing standard reagents used by students. Other rooms were equipped with feeding materials, electric mill, autoclave, water still, large drying ovens, seminar rooms, private laboratories, photographic gear, shavings storage facilities, and a refrigerator.

Teaching consisted of lectures, laboratory work, seminar, and conferences. The first course dealt with laboratory work, analysis of food and water, detection of adulterations, food product control, use the chemical methods in food laboratories and health departments. The second course covered methods of analysis of blood, urine, and tissues, especially designed to familiarise students with methods used in the study of metabolic problems. The third course focused on metabolism and diet, covering research on the field of nutrition, nutritional deficiencies, and malnutrition. The fourth course was devoted to the technique of animal experimentation. Course number five consisted of lectures and conferences on sanitary production and the handling of foodstuffs: milk, ice cream, bottled beverages, meat, baked products, canned vegetables, etc. During these courses, many industrial plants were visited.

The department had a staff of eight: professor, associate professor, two associates, three assistants, and a departmental secretary. Four attendants were employed in the care of animals and apparatus. The annual budget was $24,760 (of which $5,900 was for current expenses).

Department of the Filterable Viruses

Organised in 1922 as a part of the medical zoology department, it became independent a few years later. A general course on filterable viruses was given during the second trimester to introduce students to the filter passing agents which were responsible for so many infectious diseases. In the laboratory, students learnt methods for the isolation of filterable viruses, their biological properties, and nature of the clinical, pathological, histological, and cytological reactions of the host organism. In addition to filterable viruses, several disease-producing agents were also considered: such as rickettsia, and the tsutsugamushi disease virus.

The staff consisted of a resident lecturer, a student assistant, and a student technician. Some of the subjects under investigation included: experimental measles; varicella; diagnoses of smallpox; relations between poultry pox and vaccine; nature of infectious tumour of fowls; herpetic virus in the body of the infected host; diagnostic significance of the virus Prowazek-Halbestaedter. The budget for current expenses was $1,200 and special grants enabled research work.

Endowed with such an innovative structure, with the most modern facilities and trained staff, Johns Hopkins School became the international model school for public health expertise. Hundreds of foreign students received instruction and then imported techniques, as well as research and scientific approaches, to their home countries.

Teaching hygiene in European nations: France, Great Britain, Germany, the Netherlands, Poland, Rumania, Hungary, Yugoslavia, and Spain

The international meetings of directors of national schools of hygiene give us a rich source of information from the mid-1920s. Usually, national authorities and members of the teaching commission of the League of Nations presented reports about their respective countries, and these materials are useful for our purposes. International meetings included enquiries regarding education in hygiene and social medicine strategies in the various countries. The shaping of this network was the result of the League of Nations Health Committee decision to appoint a sub-committee to study the question of education in hygiene and social medicine in European countries, America, and Japan, and to make recommendations for courses of study which were more likely to yield the highest value in public health education both from a scientific and practical point of view.[43] The sub-committee was composed of the Frenchman Léon Bernard (chairman), Thorvald Madsen from Denmark, Witoild Chodzko from Poland, and the committee called for the assistance of suitably qualified experts. To make a unanimous tribute to the work done in this field by W.H. Welch, Director of the Public Health School of the Johns Hopkins University, 'the Committee decided to request his support by becoming a member of the Sub-Committee and thus adding the benefit of his authority and experience'.[44]

George Newman reported the situation of public health instruction in Britain.[45] He had previously published 'Recent advances in medical education in England' (1923). He focused his contribution on the efforts for improving hygiene instruction given to medical students. At the time, courses of instruction in forensic medicine, hygiene, and public health were taken with the later stages of clinical instruction. In accordance with these decisions, hygiene was systematically taught in all 27 medical schools in Great Britain.[46] Similar teaching programmes were offered at universities. Hygiene was taught in all medical schools, but only in Edinburgh, Glasgow and Aberdeen was there a full-time position for teaching hygiene. In all universities, there was a close association between hygiene and bacteriology, parasitology, and tropical medicine, and the content was included in the degree examinations in all British medical schools.

Specific instruction for health experts started in 1860, when the British Medical Association urged the General Medical Council to consider specialist qualifications and training. The 1886 Medical Act established the need for additional qualifications and specialist diplomas in sanitary science, public health, and state medicine.[47] The Local Government Act of 1888 required that medical officers in large areas should possess such diplomas. Accordingly, the General Medical Council published rules in 1889 governing diplomas and required: a) that before a candidate received a diploma in sanitary science he must be medically qualified and a period not less than 12 months should elapse between the attainment of the medical qualification and the examination for the Diploma in Public Health (DPH); b) candidates should attend practical instruction in a laboratory during six months and study outdoors with a medical officer in a large district; c) the examination should be conducted by specially qualified examiners, and should comprise laboratory work, as well as written and oral examinations.[48]

These rules remained in place until interwar years as the basis of the DPH examination. In the meantime, exceptional innovations in the knowledge and techniques took place, particularly in bacteriology. The extension of public medical services by the state and local authorities affected spheres of the social life of the population in relation to maternity, child welfare, food control, industrial employment, disease, and so forth, which substantially increased the responsibilities and enlarged the field of action of the expertise of the medical health officers.

New additional rules for the DPH were therefore deemed necessary in 1924:[49]

a) The scope of study of the diploma should be enlarged to include new subjects in social medicine regarding pathology, bacteriology, parasitology, immunology, applied chemistry and physics, epidemiology, children's diseases, maternity and infancy, tuberculosis, venereal disease, mental deficiency, occupational diseases, and food-borne disease.
b) More practical training, both administrative and sociological. The medical candidate must understand the working of sanitation in water supply, sewage systems, housing schemes, dairy farms, factories, workshops, common lodging-houses, school hygiene, meat markets, isolation hospitals, maternity homes, sanitary ports, disinfecting and cleansing stations, tuberculosis dispensaries, venereal diseases, and children's clinics.
c) The officer must be a person of some maturity and a wide clinical understanding.

The official diploma of public health training was formerly organised in all the medical schools, but under the new, more demanding rules many medical schools ceased to provide specialist instruction: a dozen of the 27 stopped teaching the courses. Specialist classes and laboratories were provided in all schools offering diploma training. The training covered a period of two years with teaching in:

- Bacteriology, parasitology, chemistry and physics in relation to public health, meteorology, and climatology.
- Principles of public health and sanitation, epidemiology and statistics, sanitary law, administration, sanitary construction, and planning.
- Clinical practice in a hospital for infectious diseases for three months.
- Practical instruction for six months under a medical officer in public health administration – including specialist instruction in maternity and child welfare, health service for school children, venereal disease, tuberculosis, industrial hygiene, and inspection and control of food.

The Diploma in Public Health (DPH) was the standard qualification required by the Ministry of Health for the appointment of medical health officers. In addition, several universities – Edinburgh, Glasgow, Birmingham, and the National University of Ireland – gave a Bachelor of Science (B.Sc.) degree in public health. The University of Liverpool also gave a master's degree in hygiene (M.H.), and the University of Durham a bachelor's degree in hygiene (B.H.). The curriculum and standard examination for these degrees was in advance of the D.P.H. standard, but the synopsis was based upon the D.P.H. curriculum. Teaching was restricted to medical staff. Examinations took place under the supervision and inspection of the General Medical Council.

With the establishment of the Institute of Medicine in association with London University, funded by the Rockefeller Foundation, a School for Public Health started official training. As already described in a previous chapter, this was the London School of Hygiene & Tropical Medicine, which was granted its Royal Charter in 1924, and moved to its present location in 1929. Both British schools of tropical medicine in London and Liverpool lost their initial clinical orientation and specialised in hygiene, public health, and prevention in tropical territories and the metropolis.

In accordance with the Rockefeller orientation, the functions of the schools were primarily instructional, although facilities for research were also afforded. The maintenance of health and the prevention of disease in temperate, as well as arctic and tropical climates was covered. The school comprised the following departments:

1   Applied physics, physiology, and principles of hygiene.
2   Chemistry and biochemistry.
3   Immunology and bacteriology.
4   Medical zoology, parasitology and comparative pathology.
5   Epidemiology and statistics.
6   Principles and practice of preventive medicine, general sanitation, and administration.

Under an agreement between the Minister of Health, the Rockefeller Foundation, and the University of London, the preliminary steps for the establishment of the School have been completed by a Transitional Executive Committee, of which the Minister of Health is Chairman.[50]

Another institution was also involved. The Ross Institute and Hospital for Tropical Diseases was opened in 1926 near Putney Heath by the Prince of Wales as a memorial to and in recognition of the work of Sir Ronald Ross. The focus of the institute was research, treatment, and prevention of tropical disease. The foundation stone was laid by the Minister of Health, Neville Chamberlain, son of the colonial secretary Joseph Chamberlain (who had been so influential in founding the original School of Tropical Medicine). Courses were largely attended by British civil servants and business people working in countries affected by tropical disease with the aim of giving individuals a basic introduction to living in tropical climates. Lectures and practical sessions were held on climatic conditions including altitude, personal hygiene, and how to prevent and treat common diseases. Due to financial problems arising after the death of Ronald Ross in 1932, the institute was incorporated into the London School, eventually to become the school's Department of Tropical Hygiene.

Wilson Jameson was appointed to the new Chair of Public Health at the London School in 1929 and became Dean in 1931 after the death of Andrew Balfour. He was also an active member of several commissions at the League of Nations. During World War Two, Jameson was the Chief Medical Officer at the

Ministry of Health and he was a decisive influence on the creation of the National Health Service through his links with the Ministry of Health and the Ministry of Education. Major Greenwood was appointed as Professor of Epidemiology and Vital Statistics. Cicely Williams was one of the first female medical students at Oxford University, subsequently studying at LSHTM in 1928–29. On joining the colonial service, she was the first woman posted to the Gold Coast (now Ghana), where in 1933 she identified *kwashiorkor*, a condition of advanced malnutrition associated with the loss of protein, usually happening when a mother weaned a toddler abruptly on the arrival of a new baby.

Non-medical health personnel should also receive specific instruction. An efficient public health administration required not only medical officers and sanitary inspectors, but also health visitors, midwives, and nurses. Specific programmes of instruction were prepared for each group. Candidates for certificate of sanitary inspector had to comply with regulations laid down by the Joint Regulation Board approved by the Ministry of Health. Candidates had to be 21 or over, have a general education, and attend a six-month course in sanitary inspector training. Examinations covered sanitary legislation, water supply, food supply, ventilation, heating and lighting, building construction, drainage and sewage, refuse disposal, prevention of disease, statistics and office procedures.

Health visitors passed an examination of the Royal Sanitary Institute approved by the Ministry of Health and received instruction at institutions approved by the Ministry (which paid grants-in-aid). Examination subjects for the diploma were elemental physiology, hygiene and sanitation, infectious and communicable diseases, maternity and child welfare, school medical service, sanitary legislation and government.

Midwives had to obtain a certificate from the government-approved Central Midwives Board. If they were certified nurses, then the course was six months; if not, the course was one-year long. They received grants-in-aid from the Ministry of Health. Their course included observing 10 deliveries and attending and nursing 20 others. Midwife candidates followed a course of lectures in physiology, anatomy and hygiene, normal and abnormal pregnancies, normal and complex deliveries, and so on. For nurses, a nursing certificate in England represented three years of hospital training as a previous condition to obtaining the diploma.

Education in hygiene and propaganda for the whole population was carefully organised by the British government. A special report was published on *Public Education in Health* and the Board of Education Syllabuses, which dealt with health teaching in elementary schools. *The Practice of Health* was used as a textbook for secondary schools. There were 109 training colleges where teachers were trained with a curriculum containing hygiene as a compulsory subject. Public education work was made by various voluntary societies.[51]

A report by B. Nocht (1925) to the League of Nations subcommittee on teaching hygiene and social medicine described the instruction of public health in Germany.[52] The course of medical study in Germany extended over a period of six years, divided into three stages: four pre-clinical terms: six clinical terms, and a year of practical medicine as a resident practitioner (*Praktikant*) in a hospital.

Students attended lectures and courses on hygiene in the second clinical period, not before the last *Studiensemestern*. There was no fixed scheme for the whole of Germany, but the state medical examination took place at the end of the second clinical stage and students could not take the practical year without passing the state examination, and the *Approbation* (state diploma) was not given until the practical training was completed. To obtain the Doctor of Medicine degree, awarded by the medical faculty independently of the state diploma, the candidate had to submit a written thesis (*dissertation*) and pass an oral examination. Subjects connected with hygiene could be selected for the thesis and oral examination. In all German universities, there were courses and lecture programmes on hygiene, bacteriology, and vaccination, and they could be included in the state examination. Courses on hygiene consisted of two terms, with a frequency of two or three lectures per week or, sometimes, five lectures per week in one term. These lectures instructed medical students on eugenics, hygienic air, climate, clothing, housing, and so on.

The president of the teaching commission of the League of Nations Health Organization, the Léon Bernard from France, contributed a report on the teaching of hygiene in the faculties and schools of medicine in France. He focused on professional instruction, without mentioning the plural initiatives in primary and secondary schools, or other public and private institutions for the general public (such as lectures given at the *Musée d'Hygiène* in Paris, social hygiene conferences at the Sorbonne, and the many others that took place in numerous French cities). The report did not deal, in fact, with the teaching of hygiene at institutions offering specialist programmes of instruction, such as sanitary technique for engineers at the Institute of Industrial Hygiene, attached to the Institute of Hygiene of the Faculty of Medicine, and others at the School of Fine Arts for Architects, those at the Faculty of Pharmacy, Schools of Nursing, and public health programmes at the Health Service of the Army for colonial troops.

Some of the medical schools in France offered hygiene teaching programmes consisting only of a cycle of lessons on the different parts of hygiene that a medical practitioner should know. In these cases, hygiene was quickly taught and students covered the entire field of hygiene. Neither the programmes, nor the number of lessons, were similar in all faculties. In Lyon and Montpellier two courses were taught in different semesters. Hygiene was taught in one semester at the medical faculties in Paris and Bordeaux, while epidemiology and social diseases occupied most of the programme. However, epidemiology and social diseases occupied a minimal place at Lille, and the content of the programme dealt with technology, labour hygiene, and legislation. The practical work revealed a common character: 'it is reduced to a small number of exercises as the chairs of hygiene do not have the necessary premises, nor the staff, nor the credits to organise real practical work.'[53]

The practical demonstrations were supplemented everywhere by visits to institutions. The most common opinion was to split the teaching of hygiene into two sections, one constituting the basic education for medical students and the other a higher education for the training of specialists in the field of medicine. After the creation by the University of Lyon of a certificate of hygiene (1905), Lille and Toulouse followed the example; and in 1920 the Faculty of Paris instituted a diploma on hygiene. Paris, Lyon, Montpellier, Bordeaux, and Algiers had instituted specialist diplomas in hygiene by 1923.

Bernard noted an even greater diversity in the programmes for the diploma of hygiene in four medical faculties. The Paris faculty aimed its diploma exclusively at medical students. Pharmacists, engineers, or architects were not accepted. The diploma was issued after passing an examination which included written tests, a report on an epidemiological survey, and oral and practical tests. Before sitting exams, the candidates needed two certificates: one in bacteriology obtained at the Institute Pasteur and another in hygiene, either from Val-de-Grâce, at the Faculty of Medicine in Paris, or that of Strasbourg. The teaching programme lasted two months and consisted of some 60 lessons covering the whole field of bacteriology, as well as laboratory manipulations. This hygiene course followed that of bacteriology and was lectured by competent experts. It included about 85 lessons during three months, supplemented by applications of chemistry to hygiene, food analysis, epidemiological research, and water bacteriology. The participants paid about 30 visits to public health institutions and campaigns. They also spent an internship period at a clinic of infectious diseases, and in health services in Paris. The total duration of the training was five months and the payment of fees was facilitated by credits allocated to the Institute of Hygiene. Grants came from the Ministry of Hygiene (30,000 Frs), the City of Paris (20,000 Frs) and the Department of the Seine (10,000 Frs).

At the Faculty of Medicine of Lyon, the diploma of hygiene was obtained after an examination that assessed two cycles of studies: a) courses and practical training on bacteriology applied to hygiene, which provided a certificate of bacteriology; b) courses, practical work, and visits on general or applied hygiene. The duration was about five months. The programme of lectures was given by medical professors and teaching staff from other faculties and higher schools, using resources and facilities of the Institute of Hygiene.

The medical faculty at Montpellier offered a degree in hygiene and a certificate in sanitary studies, open to medical doctors and students, as well as pharmacists, veterinarians, architects, engineers, and other interested people. It included lectures, practical work and visits. Hygiene courses included a basic course for future practitioners and an advanced course for specialists. In total, there were 60 lessons in hygiene and 23 lessons on legislation, geology, and chemistry. The diploma was obtained after an examination covering all the subjects in the programme. There was also a specific certificate after the examination in some of these subjects.

At the Medical Faculty in Algiers, a programme of higher education in hygiene and colonial medicine with two diplomas was instituted, one on colonial medicine and the other on hygiene. The duration of the course was four months including theoretical, practical, and clinical lectures.

The French Ministry of Public Instruction and the Ministry of Hygiene worked in 1923 on the preparation of a new project aiming to improve the training of medical students in hygiene. The project included 30 to 40 lessons on epidemiology and treatment of communicable diseases, several lectures on social diseases (tuberculosis, syphilis, alcoholism), national and international health administration, and on the hygiene problems associated with: food; water; wastewater; housing; working conditions; delivery; maternal and child health; and sanitary legislation. Practical work included demonstrations on bacteriology and notions of epidemiology, as well as chemical analysis of food, air, and water (emphasising the important role of hygiene in elementary education). In addition, there was a need in higher education to train specialists and health officials.

For appointment to public health positions, doctors who followed these activities should have been assured an advantage over those who had not followed specialist training. Therefore, the diploma was required by public health administrations for the appointment of officials. To guarantee that the diploma had a substantially equivalent value from one faculty to another, a uniform curriculum was established in terms of programme, methodology, and duration. The ministry considered it advisable, moreover, to designate the universities where courses were approved. Obviously, it was necessary to attribute to this teaching the necessary funds to ensure quality and good functioning.[54] The creation and development of the few indispensable institutes of hygiene required a financial effort which was funded by parliament.

Josephus Jitta also contributed a report on teaching public health in the Netherlands for the teaching commission of the League of Nations.[55] He explained that during the 1920s there were three state medical faculties in Holland within the universities of Leyden, Utrecht and Groningen. Exceptionally, there was also a municipal faculty in Amsterdam, governed by an 1876 act that was amended in 1922. In Leyden and Amsterdam, in addition to the chair of hygiene, there was a chair devoted to tropical medicine. The chair in Leyden was dependent on a private association for tropical medicine with its seat in Rotterdam and Leyden; while in Amsterdam it was a section for tropical hygiene of the Colonial Institute. The information contained in Jitta's report had been supplied by those responsible for teaching hygiene: Professor Eijkman in Utrecht and Professor Van Loghem in Amsterdam. Jitta arranged the structure of his report according to Léon Bernard's request for summarised national survey information on the following issues:

1   A description of the programmes of instruction, explaining which fields were taught, duration, and methods involved.
2   The organisation of chairs of hygiene and content of programmes.
3   The training programmes developed by professors of hygiene: lessons, laboratory work, and distinguished fellows.
4   System employed for endowments of chairs and selective examinations.

In Amsterdam, the programme of tropical medicine at the Institute of Tropical Hygiene (linked to the Laboratory of Hygiene at Amsterdam University) included parasitology, chemistry applied to hygiene, bacteriology, immunology, pathology, tropical hygiene, zoology, demonstrations in hospitals, practical activities in the laboratory, and field research with excursions. The course was six months long.

In Leyden, one course was on social medicine for medical practitioners, while the university organised a second course for people going to work in the Indies, including university graduates. The institute had a small hospital for tropical diseases.

A course of technical hygiene was also taught at the Polytechnic School of Delft. It was for civil engineers, electrical specialists, mining and industrial engineers, and technical chemists. Instruction in social and industrial hygiene was also taught by a medical doctor. This activity was optional.

The Dutch Board of Health organised specialist supplementary instruction for doctors in social hygiene. Examinations and diplomas were to be introduced to qualify persons seeking official positions as state, provincial, and municipal health officials, inspectors of public health, heads of health departments, industrial medical inspectors, school doctors, and other similar professional posts.

The School of Hygiene in Warsaw (Poland) was directed by Witold Chodzko. It was established for a double purpose: offering a rapid training for primary health personnel and teaching degree courses for future public health officials. It also offered specialisation courses for practitioners and medical students. The school consisted of five departments: sanitary engineering; biochemistry and nutrition; physiology and occupational health; vital statistics and epidemiology; and social hygiene. The formal inauguration of the school took place in April 1926 with the participation of the Polish Prime Minister, the Foreign Affairs Minister, and a series of distinguished foreign guests including Léon Bernard (France), Andrija Stampar and Jerislav Borcic (Yugoslavia), together with Gottfried Frey and Alfred Grotjahn (Germany).

After one decade of activity, the School of Hygiene had instructed more than 8,000 students including around 2,500 doctors. This implied providing specialised training for almost half of all the doctors practicing in Poland between the wars.[56] As in other European schools, the Warsaw school was inspired by the Johns Hopkins School of Public Health in providing specialised instruction in a broad range of disciplines related to public health. It shared the same institutional goals and structure as similar schools in Budapest and Zagreb (1926), London (1929), Madrid (1924, 1930), Prague (1926) and Athens (1930–31).[57]

A programme in microbiology in the 1920s for postgraduates was directly inspired by the Pasteur Institute's *Cours superieur de microbiologie.* A group of Polish doctors, previously Rockefeller fellows in American public health institutions, implemented the programme. All of the doctors had wide international experience. Brunon Nowakowski taught occupational medicine; Marcin Kacprzak was lecturer for vital statistics and rural hygiene; and Czeslaw Wroczynski was appointed director of the health service. Ludwik Anigstein, a parasitologist, organised and led the Museum of Hygiene along the lines of what he had seen at the London Institute of Hygiene and Tropical Medicine.[58] Hirszfeld, who had completed his medical studies in Germany, initially conceived of his department of bacteriology and experimental medicine as a Polish scientific counterpart to the Paul Ehrlich Institute in Frankfurt-am-Main.[59] K. Funk had been educated in Switzerland, Germany, and Great Britain. Witold Chodzko had spent time in Paris at the Pitié-Salpêtriere Hospital, where he worked under Joseph Babinski. Consequently, the Polish school had a wide transnational vocation and strong international links.

Infectious chronic diseases – such as tuberculosis, syphilis and alcoholism – became major social problems in Poland, once the huge post-war epidemics were under control.

Poland initiated a plan for rural health centres – which were intended to play an important role in raising health standards. Patients were treated free of charge. The centres were mainly concerned with tuberculosis prevention, infant and maternal care, but also dealt with social-sanitary problems such as alcoholism, sexually transmitted diseases, and practical questions of water supplies, nutrition, waste disposal, and building standards.

The institute realised the importance of gaining authority, prestige, and acceptance among the public and placed great emphasis on involving its scientists in public health activities, lectures, and conferences. It published several journals, such as *Medycyna doswiadczalna a spoleczna* [Experimental and Social Medicine] and *Kronika epidemiologiczna* [Chronicle of Epidemiology]. A Museum of Hygiene opened in 1925. It received some 5,000 visitors a year and helped popularise hygiene concepts.[60]

Witold Chodzko, as head of the Polish Institute and member of the Health Committee of the League of Nations, presented in 1926 to the teaching commission a report on public health training in Rumania.[61] Its text was the result of an exploratory visit initiated on May 1925, when he was received by J. Cantacuzene and visited a long list of health institutions in the country. He interviewed N.N. Saveanu, Minister for Public Health and Social Welfare; T. Gane, the Secretary-General of the Ministry; J. Bordea, Director-General for Health Services; Dr Kaminski, Assistant Director; Dr Popp, Director of Health Relief Service in the Ministry; Dr Mazincescu, Professor of Hygiene at Bucharest University; and a dozen of other medical and political authorities.[62] He also visited numerous public health institutions:

- Institute of Experimental Medicine (Professor Cantacuzene, Bucharest)
- Farm at Baneasa (annex to the Institute)
- Institute of Hygiene (Bucharest University)
- Institute and Museum of Anatomy (Bucharest University)
- State Lunatic Asylum (near Bucharest)
- Municipal slaughterhouses (Bucharest)
- Public healthcare dispensary (Rural Commune Buftea, Department Olfov)
- District Health Office (Cluj)
- Institute of General and Social Hygiene (Professor Moldovan, University Cluj)
- School of Midwifery, Obstetrical Clinic (University Cluj)
- Prostitute Control Department, State Hospital (Cluj)

Rumania had, at that time, three medical faculties at the universities of Bucharest, Jassy and Cluj. The courses were six years' long and at the end of fifth year students prepared a doctoral thesis. Bucharest had 2,000 medical students, Jassy had 900, and Cluj reached 700 students. Chairs of Hygiene were occupied at Bucharest (Professor Mazincescu), Jassy (Professor Ciuca) and Cluj (Professor Moldovan).

Public health training for medical students at Jassy University included principles of general and specialist hygiene, epidemiology and treatments for infectious diseases; methods of disinfection; land, air, and water hygiene; food hygiene; general principles of social hygiene; social diseases; and school hygiene. This course was completed with clinical instruction on infectious diseases. The state had built a hospital for infectious diseases with 150 beds.

The chair of hygiene at Bucharest had a laboratory divided into two sections: a chemical and a bacteriological section, each equipped for ten students. The hygiene course was compulsory at Bucharest and consisted of three hours per week. At Jassy, hygiene courses involved nine hours per week in the fifth year, three devoted to theory and six to practical training. At Cluj the pattern was similar. The teaching programme at Bucharest comprised technical hygiene, food hygiene, treatment for epidemics, disinfection, school hygiene, and social hygiene. There were specialist courses on urban and rural hygiene, and students wrote a monograph on health conditions at their home or summer residence. For rural areas, those surveys included a general description of the health conditions, while urban students focused on sanitation, the chief health establishments, drainage, drinking water control, slaughterhouses, preventive campaigns, health statistics, and so forth.

At Cluj there was a specialist Institute for General and Social Hygiene divided into four sections: social hygiene; preventive hygiene (including technical methods and foodstuffs control); epidemiology; and eugenics. The state contributed 162,000 lei per year. Staff included a professor, a lecturer in bacteriology, a demonstrator with two assistants, five assistants for the preparation of experiments, several laboratory assistants, and three porters. Social hygiene was taught with lectures in venereology and dermatology, paediatrics, and internal medicine. Every student at Cluj was required to spend a period of two months attached to a rural health service after passing the theoretical and practical examination in hygiene courses (this was a condition to obtain the diploma).

A new era began with the Sanitary Act of 18 December 1910.[63] The country was divided into 11 health districts, each containing between five and 14 administrative departments. Each district was under the control of a medical director who acted as the head of the area health service. A departmental medical officer coordinated various departments. There were 71 health officers covering the whole country. Each department and large town had a health council headed by the mayor and was divided into several urban and rural health districts. All officials were paid by the state (except the directors of health districts engaged in practical duties). All were under the control of the Ministry of Public Health (except those belonging to great hospital foundations and the Jewish communities).

The state maintained 11 hygiene laboratories, one for each sanitary area. They were endowed with bacteriological and chemical sections. Moreover, a Foodstuff Control Institute operated in Bucharest. The head of the health organisation in Rumania was the Minister of Health and Social Welfare, acting through a central health office or general directorate of health. The advisory organ of the ministry was composed of the director general of health, the general medical inspector of the army, 15 specialists in various branches of medicine, a chemist, a veterinary surgeon, a pharmacist, and three doctors representing respectively Transylvania, Bucovina, and Bessarabia.[64] The total budget of the Ministry of Health was 901,000,000 lei in 1925. The sum of 173,723,470 lei was devoted to disabled people and social relief, and the remainder (727,276,530 lei) for public health policies and hospitals. Public health and social welfare amounted 2.9% of the national budget, and hospitals and healthcare accounted for 2.35%.

Medical officers were divided into several categories: sanitary officers and hospital officers, the latter being divided into those attending general hospitals and those for specialist hospitals in large towns. Medical officers passed an exam after obtaining a medical degree and after having attended at least six months of lectures in hygiene.

Health agents were trained at specialist schools in Bucharest, Crailva, Galts, Jassy and Cluj. These agents complemented public health activities, and jobs were open to any citizen (aged between 18 and 20 for women, and 20 and 30 for men) holding a primary school certificate. Each school accepted 30 pupils and the lectures were given from October to June. Topics included sanitary policing, epidemiology, anatomy, physiology, and first-aid. After passing oral and written examinations, participants were appointed as provisional sanitary agents for three months for practical work in the field. They then passed a final examination and received the rank of 'health agent'.[65]

Visiting nurses were trained in several schools in Bucharest, Cluj, and Chisinau (Bessarabia). Women from the country districts had to be between 20 and 30 years old to qualify, possess a certificate of elementary studies, and pass an entrance examination. The course lasted two years and included practical training at a general hospital and Bucharest Children's Hospital. Graduates received a nurse's diploma. Visiting nurses worked in infant and children's care, as well as in campaigns against tuberculosis and epidemics. In 1926, diplomas were obtained by 327 nurses.

Another aspect was health education. Some notions of hygiene were given in all elementary, secondary, and teacher training schools. A course in popular hygiene, medicine, and pharmacy was given in the teacher training schools. This was taught by school doctors or natural science teachers using officially approved school manuals on hygiene.

Health information campaigns were managed by the health ministry within the statistics and propaganda department and under the general directorate of health. The budget in 1925 was 600,000 lei for health information campaigns, mainly spent publishing pamphlets, leaflets, posters, and announcements regarding social hygiene for schools and public welfare establishments. Other pictures and posters related to the fight against malaria, venereal diseases, and alcoholism were distributed to medical dispensaries. The ministry of education contributed to school health information, chiefly based on lectures on hygiene to children; lectures to parents on social diseases such as tuberculosis, syphilis, and alcoholism, and by giving free consultations and practical advice in schools.

The Institute of Hygiene was established in Budapest in 1909. The institute also took part in teaching activities. Hygiene was compulsory for medical students in the second doctoral exam and at the end of the tenth semester of medical studies. The instruction had an environmental orientation including: 1. History and generalities; 2. Notions about morbid influences, particularly the pathogenic organisms; 3. Infectious diseases and their treatment, immunities theory, disinfection; 4. Main infectious diseases, epidemiology, special protective measures; 5. Earth, water, atmosphere; 6. Housing, heating, ventilation, water supplies, pipes, and sewage systems; 7. Alimentation, main foodstuffs, drinking, alcoholism; 8. School hygiene and professional hygiene.

Pharmacy students received three hours per week of instruction in the winter semester. It was focused on the causes and treatment of infectious diseases, and the necessity for public hygiene. Law students received two hours a week of instruction during the winter semester, consisting of a scientific discussion about health regulations and the most important health legislation.[66] Laboratory work was devoted to the analysis of the principal foodstuffs and drinks (milk, butter, bread, wine and other alcoholic drinks), drinking water, and air. Only four places were offered for the best students, due to the lack of space and facilities.

There was a course offered for school medical officers and secondary school teachers every year during the winter semester. It included the most important chapters of general hygiene, particularly school hygiene, and sanitary examinations of air, ventilation, light, school facilities, fatigue, writing, soil research, water, and mineral poisons (mercury, arsenic, lead, and copper, etc.). Practical exercises were also included: checking ears, teeth, skin, infectious diseases, speech, deviation of the spine and other deformities, school psychiatry, and so on.

The teaching of hygiene in Hungary was explained to the League of Nations commission by B. Johan, Director of the State Hygienic Institute in Budapest.[67] Legislation passed in 1871 required that only a medical diploma was required to apply for posts as health officers. In 1883 another law required specialist training giving precedence to officers in the public health departments and those with experience as district health officers. After 1894, no doctor without a certificate could be appointed as health officer. The examination was held in two universities: Budapest and Kolozsvar, being the chairman of the examining committee the head of the Department of Hygiene and Public Health of the Ministry of the Interior. The examination included the following topics:

1   Public health and bacteriology
2   Pharmacology and toxicology
3   Mental diseases
4   Trachoma
5   Laws and regulations related to public health.

Nevertheless, no arrangements existed to provide facilities for the instruction on these subjects. New regulations were established in a ministerial order published in 1919: a certificate would not be issued before the candidate had first taken a course in public health and passed the examination. A three-month and mostly theoretical course was soon organised with a few visits to public health institutions. The curriculum included lectures on public health administration, social hygiene, campaigns against tuberculosis, venereal diseases, infant mortality, school hygiene, infectious diseases, especially trachoma, hospital administration, industrial hygiene, disinfection techniques, health insurance and meat inspection.

When the new State Institute of Hygiene was built in 1925 under the auspices of the Rockefeller Foundation these courses were stopped. The orientation changed and the new institute became equivalent to others in European countries. New courses were implemented in the new facilities for 24 students, as well as a department for training public health personnel. This department had a lecture room, a laboratory for bacteriological and chemical work, a museum, models and charts, adequate dressing rooms and toilets. The teaching material belonged to the State Institute of Hygiene and lecturers were members of staff, officials of the Ministry of Public Welfare, city health officials, university professors, and other experts. The course for public health officials lasted from January to September.

The budget for 1928 was 38,000 pengö including reasonable salaries for lecturers, and for those arranging visits and training in the field. This fee included the cost of materials, as well as travelling and living expenses for students during the course. The project implied dividing the course in two parts: the first part included theoretical and laboratory work and visits to health institutions. The second part focused on working in the field in Budapest and in a rural district, as well as practical training in the Infectious Disease Hospital for one month.[68]

In Spain, the National School of Health was established in Madrid in December 1924 on the basis of the Alfonso XIII Institute and the King's Hospital for Infectious Diseases.[69] As in many other European institutions, the main objectives were:

a)   Instructing and training a body of medical officers for the health administration.
b)   Instructing and preparing assistant medical officers, hospital attendants, disinfectors, and other subordinate staff.
c)   Teaching medical courses for architects, engineers, doctors, pharmacists and veterinaries.
d)   Creating a museum of public health to spread health education among the population.
e)   Instructing municipal health inspectors.

In 1925 the general health department took steps to complete the instruction of sanitary staff by allocating some of its budget to the creation of scholarships for studying abroad. The *Junta para Ampliación de Estudios e Investigaciones Científicas* [Board for Further Studies and Scientific Research] took on the scheme, which was reinforced and widened by foreign institutions such as the Rockefeller

Foundation. In line with that philosophy, the involvement of the Alfonso XIII National Institute of Hygiene and the King's Hospital for Infectious Diseases in the design of the future specialisation was considered paramount. The National Institute relied on suitable laboratories for teaching of microbiology, serology, disinfection, and physics and chemistry applied to hygiene. The King's Hospital guaranteed the in-depth study of all procedures relative to the fight against infection and the application of medical and social measures.[70]

The National School of Health [*Escuela Nacional de Sanidad*] was a good example of how the principles mentioned above worked in practice. Its first five years were characterised by a lack of resources.[71] The Rockefeller Foundation delegate for supervising and assessing the situation of public health in Spain, Charles Bayle, wrote critical reports – particularly in relation to laboratory expertise and staffing. His evaluation was confirmed by Francisco Murillo, General Director of Health:

> We are giving birth to a poor institution that is lacking in resources and living under the shadow of other more fortunate institutions. But it does not matter, I can see its future as a famous, prestigious school, endowed with all elements necessary to accomplish its goals.[72]

The school's first academic activities started in September 1925, one year after its official foundation. A Royal Order of 29 September 1925 accepted 12 students for training as health officers. Looking at the careers of these students, we can see that they – and thus, the national school – later became highly influential in the Spanish health administration.

In that first academic year, teaching was organised in two semesters with activities taking place at the *Instituto Nacional de Higiene Alfonso XIII* [National Institute of Hygiene], *Hospital del Rey* [King's Hospital for Infectious Diseases], *Parque Central de Sanidad* [Health Centre] and the *Ministerio de la Gobernación* [Ministry of Interior], accordingly to the following curriculum:[73]

First semester: infectious diseases and epidemiology; bacteriology and immunology.

Second semester: parasitology; chemistry and applied physics; urban and rural hygiene; health engineering and architecture; disinfection and sanitary practices; health administration, legislation, and statistics.[74]

The teaching staff had close links to the reformist group of health experts associated with the Rockefeller Foundation. Román García Durán, *Inspector General de Sanidad Exterior*, and Manuel Tapia, head of the *Hospital del Rey* and an RF fellow, taught the course in epidemiology and infectious diseases. Laboratory courses, such as bacteriology and immunology, were taught by Tapia together with Francisco Tello, head of the National Institute of Hygiene, and Federico Mestre Peón, the Spanish delegate at the European Conference on Rural Health (Budapest, 1930; Geneva, 1931). Parasitology was the responsibility of Gustavo Pittaluga, professor at the Madrid University and head of the parasitology department at the National Institute of Hygiene, as well as his pupil Sadi de Buen, malariologist and an RF fellow. Obdulio Fernández, Vice-Director of the National

Institute of Hygiene, and Serrano la Fuente, taught chemistry and physics as applied to hygiene. Responsible for teaching urban and rural hygiene were José Alberto Palanca and Francisco Becares, both RF fellows and health officers. Both also assumed great political responsibilities during the 1930s and 1940s. Eduardo Gallego and Bernardo Giner de los Ríos taught health engineering and architecture. Disinfection and practical training were coordinated by Victor Cortezo, head of the Health Centre, and Leopoldo Acosta, head of the port health service in Barcelona. Federico Mestre Peón and Francisco Becares were responsible for health legislation and health administration. Antonio Ortiz de Landázuri, one of the first RF fellows in the United States (1923–24), taught health demography and statistics.

Thus, collectively, the staff for training Spain's future health experts at the national school of health were associated with the RF. The objectives and social medicine ideology were obvious, although the material conditions and the expertise were initially poor. In the early years, the teaching staff worked without salary, receiving only the social prestige of participating in a great national project. During this provisional period, two cohorts of health officers graduated.

In 1929, just two years before the end of the monarchy and the start of a republican government, José Alberto Palanca was appointed as *Director General de Sanidad*, the main authority in the field of health policies. At the time, he was in the United States as an RF fellow, and the American foundation probably stood behind his appointment. Yet, it is surely not coincidental that shortly after Palanca was appointed director-general of public health, a Royal Decree of 12 April 1930 established new regulations for the national school of health that meant a re-foundation along the lines promoted in various European countries by the RF and the LNHO. The 1930 regulation made the school an independent institution; henceforth, the technical direction, programmes, practical training, internal organisation, selection of students, institutional relations, and budget management were decided exclusively by the school's own administrators.[75] This administrative independence, together with an independent budget, enabled the school's leaders to build an institution that focused on the health needs of Spanish society and, at the same time, reach European standards. Pittaluga's contribution was essential because of his national and international reputation (he was a member of the International Board for the Teaching of Hygiene and Preventive Medicine and an active member of several expert commissions of the League of Nations).

The National School of Health, together with the National Institute of Hygiene, became the main institutions for the training of health experts and for the implementation of health policies in Spain. Given their close links to state policy making, a debate arose as to their relationship with medical faculties, for it was recognised that 'a solid health culture' among doctors, medical students, and other health experts required at least a modicum of institutional and professional cooperation. The objectives laid out in the Royal Decree were much more ambitious than previous regulations and close to the present concept of public health. The school was expected to fulfil a series of targets:

1   Train health officers, i.e. experts in hygiene, social, and preventive medicine.
2   Conduct complementary courses related to applied medicine.
3   Train experts in school hygiene.
4   Create a museum of health as an instrument of public education.
5   Establish a public health board for nurses and train them to be public health visitors.
6   Promote scientific research in public health matters, epidemiology, and microbiology as applied to hygiene, statistics, and demography.
7   Publish annals, journals, and proceedings.
8   Create a central health library.

This comprehensive programme and the new mentality of social medicine produced a considerable overhaul of the school's curriculum. The number of subjects was expanded and the role of experimental laboratory courses and practical field-work was expanded as an important supplement to lectures.[76] In 1931–32 the future health officers were required to sit twelve subjects:

Bacteriology, immunology, and serology.

Food and nutrition hygiene, and bromatology.

Health statistics and demography.

General epidemiology and epidemiological techniques.

Infectious diseases and their clinical treatment.

Parasitology and tropical diseases.

Public and private general hygiene.

Social medicine and school hygiene.

Labour, industrial, and professional hygiene.

Health engineering and urban hygiene.

Health administration and international health.

Museology, iconography, and public awareness.

The National School of Health and the National Institute of Hygiene brought together a group of young professionals who had become public health experts mostly in foreign institutions, thanks to grants from the Spanish government and the Rockefeller Foundation. Marcelino Pascua, Antonio Oller, and Enrique Carrasco Cadenas, respectively professors in health statistics and demography, labour hygiene, and food and nutrition, had received a solid instruction at University College London, the Johns Hopkins School of Public Health, and the Industrial Workers Hospital at Kandersteng and Mitholz (Switzerland). Antonio Ortiz de Landázuri, professor of epidemiology and epidemiological techniques, had been an RF fellow and was the author of Spain's official reports submitted to the *International Health Yearbooks*. His collaborator in this work was Francisco Ruiz de Morote, an RF fellow with a doctorate in public health from Johns Hopkins. Lectures on infectious diseases were taught by Manual Tapia, an RF fellow leading the National Hospital for Infectious Diseases, and Juan Torres Gosp, who had studied in Germany with a grant from the *Junta de Ampliación de Estudios* (Spanish Board for Further Studies). Jimena de la Vega, who had studied in Berlin, Vienna, and Hamburg, was appointed to the chair in labour, industrial, and professional hygiene.

Moreover, many staff also occupied leading positions in other health institutions, which confirmed the school's role in the national network of health experts. Antonio Ruiz Falcó, teaching bacteriology, serology and immunology, was simultaneously head of the *Instituto de Biología y Sueroterapia*. José Sánchez Verdugo was in charge of statistics at the *Dirección General de Sanidad;* José Germain, a well-known expert in experimental psychology, led the mental hygiene section at the *Dirección General de Sanidad* and was an active member of the International Committee of Mental Hygiene in Industry, as well as of the International Association of Psychotechnology, and the International Committee of Tests; José Estellés Salarich, professor for cinematography and iconography, also held the office of *Inspector General de Sanidad*. And finally, as noted earlier, the professor for general public and private hygiene, José Alberto Palanca, was appointed Spain's Director General of Health in 1929, and was later head of the health services under Franco.

Information on the number of applicants for admission to the National School of Health in Madrid confirms that it appealed to young doctors. During the academic term 1931–32, 267 applicants vied for the 40 positions; the following year 74 applicants sought 20 places. As school director, Pittaluga noted, preventive and social medicine was clearly a popular speciality among doctors, and the title of health officer and incorporation into the National Health Board were attractive career options.

During the early 1930s, while Marcelino Pascua, the school's professor of statistics, was the General Director of Health under the first socialist government of the Spanish Republic, the National School of Health was assigned a new mandate and given more solid financial support including funding for teaching assistants. However, this situation was short-lived. In 1934 the newly installed conservative coalition government carried out a policy of financial retrenchment that resulted in a reorganisation of Spain's health administration. This had drastic consequences for the National School of Health. It lost its autonomous position and was integrated into the National Institute of Hygiene as the Section for Health Studies.[77]

The Spanish Civil War severely undermined the training of public health experts in the country. The teaching staff of what had been the National School of Health were much reduced in number by the effects of exile, murder, and imprisonment.[78] During the war years only a few individual courses on bacteriology, malariology, and parasitology took place, a situation prolonged until 1948, when regular courses restarted for *Diplomados en Sanidad*.[79] Nevertheless, the scientific and academic level was far removed from the level reached in the early 1930s. Of the well-trained staff of those years, only F. Ruíz Morote and José Román Manzanete remained, teaching respectively epidemiology and microbiology, and serology and parasitology. Social medicine and the role of public health experts had changed greatly by then, and Spain was isolated under an authoritarian regime.

International initiatives: courses in London and Paris

During the period of institutionalisation and expansion of national schools of hygiene, the Health Committee of the League of Nations prompted two international courses of hygiene devoted to European experts in public health. These took place in Paris and London in 1927.[80] The Paris course was held at the Hygiene Laboratory of the Medical Faculty and included a wide range of activities in other facilities and institutions. The content of the programme shows an ambitious updating of public health and social medicine issues with the participation of most leading European countries. The course lasted almost two months from 17 January until 5 March 1927 and included the following lectures, seminars, and activities:

17 January: Léon Bernard, The evolution of hygiene and preventive medicine in relation to health officers and medical bodies.

18 January: M. Stouman: Present distribution of epidemics (I)
P. Saiki: The feeding metabolism (I)
Visit to the *Institut prophylactique antivénéreen* (Paris)

19 January: M. Stouman: Present distribution of epidemics (II)
P. Saiki: The feeding metabolism (II)
Meeting-conference: Hygiene Laboratory

20 January: P. Bordet: General principles of immunology
Meeting-conference: Hygiene Laboratory

21 January: M. Schlossman: Hospital care for the first age (I)
M. Saiki: The feeding metabolism (III)
Meeting-conference: Hygiene Laboratory

22 January: M. Schlossman: Hospital care for the first age (II)
Visit to the *Institut Supérieur de la Vaccine et contrôle des vaccines*
(Paris)

24 January: M. Calmette: Specific vaccination against tuberculosis
Meeting-conference: Hygiene Laboratory

25 January: Pasteur Hospital
Meeting-conference: Hygiene Laboratory

26 January: M. Besredka: Specific vaccination against cholera, dysentery, and typhoid. Oral vaccination. Institute Pasteur

27 January: Visit to the *Cité Jardins de la Compagnie du Nord* (Terguier, Aisne)

28 January: M. Chennevier: Hospital care and hygiene
Meeting-conference: Hygiene Laboratory

29 January: Visit to the *Organisation obstétricale de prophylaxie sociale anti-vénéreenne et anti-tuberculeuse* (Paris)
Meeting-conference: Hygiene Laboratory

31 January: M. Levaditi: Anti-variolique vaccine
M. Funk: Vitamins (I)
M. Thierry: Theory and practice of disinfection (I)
Meeting-conference: Hygiene Laboratory

1 February: M.R. Debré: Specific prophylaxis of rubella
M. Funk: Vitamins (II)
Visit to school health centres, activity by the society 'L'Hygiène par l'exemple'.

2 February: M. James: Tropical diseases in Europe (I)
M. Gunn: General considerations about public health administration (I)

3 February: Visit to St. Louis Hospital, General Hospital, and Nursery of Dr Jules Renault Museum (Paris)

M. Gunn: General considerations about public hygiene (II). Respective value of different types of public services.

4 February: M. James: Tropical diseases in Europe (II)
Visit to the Institute Pasteur.

5 February: M. Chailley Bert: Physical education
M. Winslow: Drinking water
Visit to the disinfection centre of Ville de Paris

7 February: M. Gilbert: Health control labour
M. Winslow: Water sterilisation
Visit to service of mental prophylaxis of children

8 February: M. Debré: Specific prophylaxis in scarlet fever
M. Carozzi: Organisation of industrial work and several factors (I)
M. Gougerot: Anti-venereal prophylaxis (film and lecture)

9 February: M. Winslow: Depuration of black water
M. Carozzi: Organisation of industrial work and several factors (II)
M. Debré: Visit to laboratory of sero-prophylaxis of rubella

Meeting-conference: Hygiene Laboratory
M. Winslow: About ventilation

10 February: Visit to hospital centre for care and prophylaxis of tuberculosis. Dispensary Léon Bourgeois, Hospitalization quartier, social services, Laënnec Hospital
Sewage services
M. Winslow: Milk

11 February: M. Ramon: Diphtheria and Tetanus Specific prophylaxis
M. Carozzi: Industrial work organisation and factors involved
M. Winslow: Visiting nurses and public health

12 February: M. Velghe: Worker housing
M. Sand: Popular teaching of hygiene

14 February: Visit to the sanatorium anti-tuberculosis of Bligny (Paris)

15 February: M. Winslow: Individual hygiene
M. Mackenzie: School age hygiene (I) Film on social hygiene organisation

16 February: Visit to factory guided by work inspectors
M. Mackenzie: School age hygiene (II)
Meeting-conference: Hygiene Laboratory

17 February: Visit to Loing wellsprings (providing water to Paris)

18 February: M. Heyermans: Municipal administration of hygiene
M. Lepine: Prophylaxis of mental diseases
Meeting-conference: Hygiene Laboratory

19 February: Visit to Centre de la Forté, prophylaxis of tuberculosis through feeding

21 February: M. Pittaluga: Epidemiology from a biological perspective (I)
M. Madsen: Specific prophylaxis of whooping cough
Visit to Institute of Radium

22 February: M. Pittaluga: Epidemiology from a biological perspective (II)
M. Madsen: Season cycle of epidemics
M. March: Statistical methodology (I)
Meeting-conference: Hygiene Laboratory

23 February: M. Pittaluga: Epidemiology from a biological perspective (III)
M. Madsen: Standardisation of serum and biological products
Visit to dispensary of Vanves, a complete dispensary for social hygiene

24 February: M. March: Statistical methodology (II)
L. Bernard: Scientific principles of the fight against anti-tuberculosis
Visit to the State Statistical Office (Paris)

25 February: M. March: Statistical methodology (III)
M. Methorst: Applied statistics to demography and public health (I)
M. Methorst: Applied statistics to demography and public health (II)

26 February: M. Methorst: Applied statistics to demography and public health (III)
L. Bernard: Social prophylaxis of tuberculosis
Meeting-conference: Hygiene Laboratory
M. Gini: Sanitary problems related to migrations

28 February: Visit to several factories
M. Hahn: Infectious diseases permanent organisations

1 March: M. Kuhn: Danish example for health care insurance (I)
L. Bernard: Legal anti-tuberculosis measures
Meeting-conference: Hygiene Laboratory

2 March: M. Kuhn: Danish example for healthcare insurance (I)
M. Forestier: Principles of urbanism
Visit to spreading fields at Achèroc

3 March: M. Boudreau: Rural hygiene administration
M. Pottevin: International Sanitary Conventions
Visit to Paris water supplies: chlorination and factory ozonisation

4 March: M. Foramitti: Social insurances and preventive medicine (I)
L. Rajchman: The League of Nations Health Organization
Visit to the National Office for Social Hygiene established with funds of the Rockefeller Foundation at the Ministry of Health

5 March.   M. Foramitti: Social insurances and preventive medicine (II)
L. Bernard: International sanitary cooperation

The list of lectures and institutes visited shows practically all visits were related to social medicine. The political dimension of the event attracted not only experts and lecturers, the following participants attended the International Course of Hygiene as representatives of their countries:[81]

Bulgaria: Athanase Nedeff, departmental doctor at Bourgas.
Estonia: Hans Alver, departmental doctor at Hapsal.
Greece: Kostis Charitakis, Head of Social Hygiene Service, Ministry of Health, Athens.
Michel Boyadgis, Central Service, Ministry of Health, Athens.

Hungary:	Arthur Pollerman, Advisor, Ministry of Social Prevention, Head of the Centre for Social Propaganda, Budapest. Charles Grosch, Advisor, Ministry of Social Prevention, Budapest.
Lithuania:	Atanas Jurgelionis, Head of the Laboratory of Army Hygiene.
Luxembourg:	Pierre Schmol, Associate Doctor at Bacteriological State Laboratory.
Paraguay:	Dr Melgarejo, National Department of Hygiene and Public Care.
Poland:	B. Ostromecki, Head of Health Department of Kielce District.
Rumania:	De Spiru, General Health Inspector, Arad Region. V. Popesco, General Health Inspector, Galata Region.
Kingdom of the Serbs, Croats & Slovens:	Y. Kouchlech, Epidemiologist at Central Institute of Hygiene, Belgrade.
Czechoslovakia:	F. Skacelik, Public Health Inspector, Ministry of Hygiene and Physical Education, Prague. F̄.R. Ziel, Departmental Health Inspector, Ministry of Hygiene and Physical Education, Prague.
USSR:	Dr Nikolski, Head of the Prophylaxis Section, Public Health Department, North Caucase. D̄r D. Livchitz, People's Commissar Public Health of White Russia.

The international network was very active. A second International Course of Public Health took place the same year in London (1927). All lectures were at the Society of Medical Officers of Health and the programme was as follows:

M. Taute: 'The development of the administration and practice in public health in Germany'.

W.W.C. Topley, London School of Hygiene, University of London: 'Herd immunity', who also chaired a symposium on immunology.

William Hamer. Formerly Medical Officer of Health, County of London: 'London Epidemics of 250 years ago and today: the contrasts and resemblances'.

S.F. Dudley, Professor of Pathology, Royal Naval College: 'Immunology: field observations'.

Carl Browning, Pathological Institute, University of Glasgow: 'The virus and the host: their respective parts in the spread of infectious disease'.

Andrew Balfour, Director of the London School of Hygiene: 'Education of medical officers for service in the tropics: I. Tropical medicine. II. Tropical hygiene'.

J.J. Buchan, Medical Officer of Health, Bradford: two lectures on 'Industrial hygiene'.

K. Stouman, Health Section, League of Nations: two lectures on 'The geographical distribution of epidemic diseases'.

B. Nocht: Director of the Institute of Tropical Hygiene, Hamburg: 'The present position of chemotherapy from the clinical point of view'.

Dr Schrubsall coordinated a visit to Institutions for Mentally Defective Persons at Epsom.

EP Cathcart, Department of Physiology, University of Glasgow: 'Nutrition: the qualitative aspect'. He also coordinated a symposium on nutrition.

H. Emerson, Columbia University, United States:

> 'Heart diseases: A public health problem'.
>
> 'Epidemiology of other than the communicable diseases'.
>
> 'Public health and private responsibility'.
>
> 'Experience of New York City with diphtheria'.

E. Mapother, Kings College Hospital & Maudsley Hospital: 'Mental hygiene'. Followed by a visit to Maudsley Hospital.

J.F. Buchan, Medical officer of health in Willesden: 'Maternity and child welfare centres at Willesden' and a further visit to Maternity and Child Welfare Centres at Willesden.

A. Daley, Medical Officer of Health, Hull: two lectures on 'Public education in health'.

U. Friedmann, Medical School Officer: 'Epidemiology of the infectious disease of childhood' and visit to schools.

F.C. Schrubsall, Senior Medical Officer: 'The problem of the abnormal child' and 'Special schools' followed by visit to schools for physically defective children.

R.A. Lyster, County Medical Officer of Health, Hampshire: 'Training of the medical officer of health and his staff' (two lectures).

C.J. Thomas, Senior Medical Officer 'The medical inspection and treatment of school children'.

H.R. Kenwood, Emeritus Professor of Hygiene University of London, two lectures in 'Rural hygiene' and further visit to points of interest in the county in Bedfordshire.

F.G. Boudreau, Health Section, League of Nations: 'The activities of the Health Section, League of Nations'.

G.S. Buchan, Senior Medical Officer, Ministry of Health, London: 'The position of certain preventable diseases in relation to public health administration'.

G.H. de Paulo-Souza, Director Institute Public Health, Sao Paulo: 'Modern practice of preventive medicine in a new country'.

G.M. Fyfe, Medical Officer of Health, St. Andrews: 'A scheme for cooperation between general practitioners and the public health department'.

Participants in the London international course also visited the Museum of the Institute of Hygiene. The two international courses in Paris and London (1927) for public health experts aimed to promote international cooperation in technical issues related to health problems, such as bacteriological and serological methods, the recording of epidemiological data, agreements about standards of vaccines and so on. Medical officers from 20 different nations, mostly European, attended these courses and then participated in a practical training tour in many European countries.[82]

The great failure: *École Internationale d'Hautes Études d'Hygiène* [International School of Advanced Studies in Hygiene]

After the celebration of international courses for public health experts in Paris and London in 1927, and subsequent meetings of directors of national schools in Dresden and Paris, in November 1930, the Health Committee of the League of Nations reported to the League Council a proposition of the French government to establish an International School of Advanced Studies in Hygiene [*École Internationale d'Hautes Études d'Hygiène*] under the auspices of the League of Nations.[83] The project was undoubtedly shaped with the complicity of all the participants. Therefore, the Council of the League of Nations initially accepted the proposal and invited the Health Organization and the Secretariat to initiate a technical assessment of the project, based on the details delivered by the French government and on its own considerations. The report was to be later submitted again to the Council for a final decision. The Health Committee considered that the future *École Internationale d'Hautes Études d'Hygiène* would complete and implement the programme shaped during the several meetings of directors of national schools of public health.

As a consequence of the 1930 Paris Conference and the positive effects of an international agreement on public health policies, the French government made a proposal for 'The Creation of an International School of Advanced Studies in Hygiene in Paris'.[84] The proposal discussed all the necessities and demands, the technical organisation, the teaching staff, number and type of students, general programme of instruction, administrative organisation, and financial needs. The project was sent to the International Health Division of the Rockefeller Foundation after having been previously approved by the Council of the League of Nations. Bernard's report was accompanied by a letter from the French Government to the

President of the League's Council, containing an annex entitled 'Statutes of the International School of Advanced Health Studies'. Léon Bernard, as an expert and delegate of the French government at the League, developed the role of commentator. Rajchman requested the opinion and agreement of the directors of the national schools of public health, but there is no reference to such an agreement in the document. No other archival documents, neither at the Rockefeller Archives, nor the League of Nations Archives, discuss this issue.

When the Rockefeller Foundation received the proposal, the IHD authorities requested the confidential opinion of a series of professors and experts in public health. They also requested the opinion of Hampstead Laboratories and Milbank Memorial Fund. The response was unanimously positive towards the initiative. The political process started when the Council of the League of Nations passed the proposal on 24 September 1930, the health section issued a draft by Léon Bernard, stating the commitment of the French government to the creation of an International School of Advanced Studies in Hygiene with the support of the Rockefeller Foundation.

Teaching was to be in French, and the school would have been endowed with permanent professorships, together with a certain number of prominent French and foreign professors. It is easy to assume that the list of professors would coincide with the elite of the very active transnational network. Students were to be medical doctors, specialised in hygiene, health officers, health administrators, and future leaders of national health services and national schools of hygiene. They would have received grants from the League of Nations, from their governments, and other institutions.

The teaching activities at the International School would have consisted of lectures, seminars and practical activities. The programme of lectures had three parts: comparative general hygiene; advances in hygiene and related fields; and international sanitary cooperation.[85]

A　Comparative general hygiene included:

General organisation: economy, political and social foundations of hygiene.
Public hygiene in its different modalities.
Social hygiene.
Rural hygiene.
Labour and industrial hygiene.
Medical care and hospitals.
Housing and urbanism.
Ports, navigation, and quarantines.
Sanitary technique.
Laboratory in relation with public health.
Health education for the population.

B　Advanced studies in hygiene and related fields: physical sciences, chemistry, biology, sociology, human geography in relation with public health, legislation and administration regarding national and international sanitary legislation.

C   International sanitary cooperation.

Hygiene movement worldwide.
International sanitary conferences and conventions.
The League of Nations work in hygiene.
The *Office International d'Hygiène Publique.*
The work of private associations in public health.

The school project provided two types of courses. A general one containing the fundamentals and other specialist courses for specific demands. The general course was a six-month period of lectures, seminars, practical training, and travel.

In accordance with the French government's proposal, the school would become an instrument for the League of Nations, although free from any legal responsibility. From a financial perspective, the French state assumed the requirements for its establishment, maintenance, and functioning, although the Health Organization could contribute fellowships to improve resources. Despite the direct involvement of the League of Nations, the director was to be appointed by the French government and had to be a prominent French figure in public health.

The first version of this project was approved by the Council of the League of Nations in 24 September 1930. Its goals were explicitly, under the auspices of the Health Organization of the League of Nations, to become the leading permanent institution for the teaching of public health, reinforcing interchange programmes promoted by the League, and financed by the Rockefeller Foundation.[86] It would give a wider view to programmes at the national schools of hygiene and prepare leaders for national health administrations, update knowledge and techniques for health experts, administrators, and inspectors.

The International School was to be managed by an administrative board composed of members of the Health Committee of the League. The international members accepted the project, but the project was still not implemented by 1937. The French senate finance committee finally rejected the funding and facilities for the project on 7 April 1938.

On 29 June, 1939, L. Rajchman visited the Rockefeller Foundation at New York together with Jean Monnet (one of the founding fathers of the European Union project). Rajchman explained that the project for an international school of hygiene in Paris had been stopped by the French senate finance committee. Caillaux, chairman of the finance committee and Minister of Finance, said the French government could provide FF 1,000,000 for maintenance, with the question remaining open as to whether the new school was to be located at Suresnes. An important detail is that the international school that Rajchman had in mind would not be for medical officers but for directors of schools of hygiene. It would open six months a year with field studies and facilities for applying ideas in various domains. Rajchman was thinking of an international faculty, one group of which would serve from two to six months, and another on a three-year appointment to develop a specialist field. The estimation was that FF 2,000,000 were needed for the next two years to bring in lecturers and provide scholarships for participants. A meaningful part of the funds had to be allocated by the participant governments.[87]

However, the war years introduced significant changes. On 6 April 1942, a letter from S. Deutschman, former officer at the International Labour Organisation (ILO) to George K. Strode, Associate Director IHD, RF stated:

> I have received a letter from Dr Biraud dated 16 February containing a paragraph which I think may interest you: '*En France une loi vient de créer à Paris un Institut National d'Hygiène sur le plan que vous connaissez; puisque c'est celui dejà envisagé il y a un an. La direction en a été donnée par décret au Prof. André Chevallier, professeur de pharmacologie à Marseille, vu jadis avec le Dr. Strode. Vous devinez ce que pense le Prof. Parisot qui a rejoint son post à Nancy...*'[88] This was not the only unexpected news, as he also explained that: 'The Epidemiological Intelligence Service is carrying on its work despite the absence of data from the Far Eastern countries. The Singapore branch closed down on 20 January 1942, and Dr Park left for Australia. The Section is still receiving a number of requests for technical information from various health administrations. Dr Gautier and Dr Biraud recently wrote a short report on the nutrition situation in Europe intended for a study by Mr. Loveday at Princeton.[89]

World War Two radically changed the landscape of the international public health structure built during the previous decades.

Notes

1 Bernard, L. 'Report on the Conference held at the Inauguration of the Budapest and Zagreb Schools of Public Health', Geneva: LONA, C.H.661, October 27, 1927, pp. 8–9.
2 Chodzko, W. 'Collaboration between the different Schools of Hygiene.' Geneva: LONA, C.H.645, 1927.
3 Pelc, H. 'Preliminary Report on Programmes of Schools of Public Health', Geneva: LONA, C.H.623, 1927; Pelc, H. 'Supplementary Report on Programmes of Schools of Public Health', Geneva: LONA, C.H.623 (a), 1927.
4 Chodzko, W. 'The Programme of Courses at the Polish State School of Hygiene.' Geneva: LONA, C.H.627, 1927.
5 Stampar, A. 'The Zagreb School of Hygiene', Geneva: LONA, C.H.417, 1927, p. 2; Stampar, A. 'Supplementary note relating to training at the School of Hygiene, at Zagreb.' Geneva: LONA, C.H.417 (a), 1927.
6 Chodzko, W. 'The Methods of Recruiting Students for Schools of Hygiene.' Geneva: LONA, C.H. 628, 1927.
7 Chodzko, W. 'The Programme of Courses.' (1927), pp. 2–3.
8 Ibidem.
9 Ibidem.
10 Johan, B. 'Relations between Hygienic Institutes in various countries and possible means of cooperation.' Geneva: LONA, C.H.644, 1927.
11 Chodzko, W. 'Collaboration between the different Schools of Hygiene' (1927).
12 Barona, 'The Rockefeller Foundation' (2015).
13 *Société des Nations*, Genève: Société des Nations, 1931, p. 18.

14 LONA holds a series of documents: C.H.238, C.H.362, C.H.277, C.H.286 and C.H.867.
15 Bayley, Ch. 'Public Health in Spain' 1926, Terrytown, New York: RAC, Record Group: 1.1. Projects, Series 795 Spain, folder 1.
16 Barona, 'The Rockefeller Foundation' (2015).
17 Barona, 'The Rockefeller Foundation' (2015).
18 Bernard, L. 'Report on the Conference held at the Inauguration of the Budapest and Zagreb Schools', (1927).
19 Bernard, L. 'Committee on the Teaching of Hygiene. Report on the Teaching of Hygiene in Europe by . . .' Geneva: LONA, C.H.243, 1927.
20 'Report on the Conference on Schools of Public Health held at Budapest and Zagreb from September 29 to October 4, 1927', Geneva, LONA, C.H.659, 1927.
21 Report on the Conference on Schools, 1927, p. 8.
22 Ibidem.
23 'Reports on Schools of Public Health', Geneva: LONA, Doc. C.H.873 and 865.
24 Balfour, 'Public Health Training in the USA', Geneva: LONA, Doc. C.H.870, 1930.
25 Vacek, B.; Pelc, H. 'Report on teaching public health in Prague', Geneva: LONA, Doc. C.H.871, 1930.
26 Kacprzak, M. 'The School of Public Health in Warsaw', Geneva: LONA, Doc. C.H.872.
27 Stampar, A. 'The School of Public Health in Zagreb', Geneva: LONA, Doc. C.H.873 and 865, 1930.
28 Johan, B. 'Teaching Public Health in Hungary', Geneva: LONA, Doc. C.H.873 and 865, 1930.
29 Prausnitz, C. 'Report on Teaching Public Health in Europe', Geneva: LONA, Doc. C.H.873 and 865, 1930.
30 Barona Vilar, J.L. 'Public Health Experts and Scientific Authority'. In Andresen, A.; Hubbard, W.; Ryymin, T. (eds) *International and Local Approaches to Health and Health Care*, Oslo: Novus Press, 2010, pp. 31–48.
31 Prausnitz, C. 'Report on teaching public health in Europe', Geneva: LONA, Doc. C.H.880.
32 Ibidem.
33 *The School of Hygiene and Public Health of the Johns Hopkins University*, Baltimore: The American Journal of Hygiene Monographic Series, 1926.
34 'The School of Hygiene and Public Health' (1926), p. 15.
35 'The School of Hygiene and Public Health' (1926), pp. 15–17.
36 'The School of Hygiene and Public Health' (1926), p. 18.
37 Ibidem.
38 Ibidem, pp. 19–22.
39 Ibidem, pp. 26–28.
40 Ibidem, p. 30.
41 Ibidem, p. 31.
42 Ibidem, pp. 39–40.
43 Bernard, 'Committee on the Teaching of Hygiene' (1927).
44 Ibidem.
45 Newman, G. 'Health Education in Great Britain', Geneva: LONA, C.H.362, 1925; 'Memorandum on the Organization and Functions of the Ministry of Health (England and Wales)'. Ministry of Health, March 1925, Geneva: LONA, 123/47764/26249, 1925.
46 Newman, 'Health Education in Great Britain' (1925), p. 1.
47 Newman, 'Health Education in Great Britain' (1925), p. 2.
48 Ibidem, pp. 2–3.
49 Ibidem.
50 Wilkinson, L.; Hardy, A. *Prevention and Cure: the London School of Hygiene & Tropical Medicine: a 20th century quest for global public health*, London: Kegan Paul Limited, 2001, p. 3.

51 Newman, 'Health Education in Great Britain' (1925), p. 8.
52 Nocht, B. 'Report on the academic teaching of Hygiene and social medicine at German universities, technical high schools and academies for social hygiene.' Geneva: LONA, C.H.277, 17 March, 1925.
53 Bernard, L. 'Rapport sur l'enseignement de l'Hygiène en France', Geneva: LONA, C.H.134, 1923, p. 4.
54 Ibidem, p. 13.
55 Jitta, J. 'The Teaching of Hygiene in the Netherlands', Geneva: LONA, C.H.286, April 3, 1925.
56 Balinska, M.A. 'The National Institute of Hygiene and Public Health in Poland 1918–1939'. *Social History of Medicine*, 9, 1996, p. 442.
57 Ibidem.
58 'Letter from L. Rajchman to C. Weynon, 9 April 1923', LONA, 12B 27967/26533, 1923.
59 Balinska, 'The National Institute of Hygiene', p. 440.
60 Ibidem, p. 443.
61 Chodzko, W. 'Report on Public Health Training in Roumania', presented by . . . Geneva: LONA, C.H.475, June 2, 1926.
62 Chodzko, 'Report on Public Health Training in Roumania . . .' 1926.
63 Chodzko, 'Report on Public Health Training in Roumania . . .' 1926.
64 Kaminski, Dr, 'The Health Organization of Roumania, Bucharest', 1923.
65 Chodzko, 'Report on Public Health Training in Roumania', 1926, p. 15.
66 Chodzko, 'Report on Public Health Training in Roumania', 1926, p. 8.
67 Johan, B. 'The Training of the Public Health Officers in Hungary', Geneva: LONA, C.H.630, 1927.
68 Ibidem.
69 Escuela Nacional de Sanidad. Reglamento y Programas, Madrid: Imprenta José Molina, 1926.
70 *Escuela Nacional de Sanidad* (1926), pp. 112–113. Navarro García, R. *Historia de las Instituciones Sanitarias Nacionales*, Madrid: Instituto de Salud Carlos III, 2001, pp. 50–57.
71 Barona Vilar, J.L.; Bernabeu-Mestre, J. *La Salud y el Estado. El movimiento sanitario internacional y la administración española (1851–1945)*, Valencia: Publicaciones de la Universidad de Valencia, 2008.
72 'Escuela Nacional de Sanidad' (1926), p.112.
73 'Escuela Nacional de Sanidad' (1926), p. 36.
74 'Exposición que precede al RD de 12 de abril de 1930, donde se establecen las justificaciones para la elaboración de un nuevo Reglamento de la Escuela Nacional de Sanidad', Madrid: *Gaceta*, 22 April, 1930.
75 Pittaluga, G. *La constitución de la Escuela Nacional de Sanidad*, Madrid: Publicaciones de la Escuela Nacional de Sanidad, 1930.
76 'Resumen de la labor realizada por la Escuela Nacional de Sanidad durante el cuso 1931–1932', *Revista de Sanidad e Higiene Pública*, 8:1, 1933, pp. 66–70.
77 Bernabeu-Mestre, J. La salud pública que no va poder ser. José Estellés Salarich (1896–1990): una aportació valenciana a la sanitat espanyola contemporània, València: Consell Valencià de Cultura (Serie Minor, 62), 2007.
78 Bernabeu-Mestre, Josep, 'La utopía reformadora de la Segunda República: la labor de Marcelino Pascua al frente de la Dirección General de Sanidad, 1931–1933', *Revista Española de Salud Pública*, 74, 2000, pp. 1–13.
79 *Memoria de la Dirección General de Sanidad*, Madrid: Ministerio de la Gobernación, 1943–1945; *Memoria de la Dirección General de Sanidad*, Madrid: Ministerio de la Gobernación, 1948.
80 'Cours internationale d'Hygiène organisé par le Commité d'Hygiène de la Société des Nations à la Faculté de Médecine de Paris', Geneva: LONA, C.H./E.P.S./123, 192.

81 'Liste des auditeurs du Cours International d'Hygiène organisé par l'Institut d'Hygiène de la Faculté de Médecine de Paris sur l'initiative et avec le concours du Comité d'Hygiène de la Société des Nations.' Geneva: LONA, 13/1/1927, C.H./E.P.S./124, 1927.

82 'Grant for the maintenance of a system of interchange of public health personnel on an international scale'. Terrytown, New York, RAC, RG1.1. Series 100, Box 21, Folder 175, 1930, p. 3.

83 'Création à Paris, sous les auspices de la Société des Nations, d'un Centre International de Hautes Études d'Hygiène', Geneva: LONA, C.535.1930.III, 1930; 'Création à Paris d'une École Internationale de Hautes Études d'Hygiène. Rapport du Comité d'Hygiène au Conseil de la Société des Nations relative à la proposition du gouvernement français', Geneva: LONA, C.589.1930.III, 1930.

84 Bernard, L. 'Report by Prof . . . on behalf of the Sub-Committee appointed to examine the French Government Proposal for the Creation of an International School of Advanced Health Studies at Paris', Terrytown, New York: RAC RG 6.1, series 1.1, box 38, folder 466, 1930.

85 'Création à Paris, sous les auspices de la Société des Nations' (1930).

86 Barona, 'The Rockefeller Foundation . . .', (2015).

87 Terrytown, New York: RAC, RG 1.1, series 100, box 22, folder 181 (1938–1941).

88 'Letter from S. Deutschman to George K. Strode', Terrytown, New York: RAC, 6 April 1942, RG 1.1, series 100, box 22, folder 182, 1942–1944.

89 'Letter from S. Deutschman to George K. Strode' (1942–1944).

7   Final comments and conclusions

This book is the result of a historical analysis to discover how specific transnational powers developed an extensive programme of institutionalisation and expansion of public health during the interwar years. The starting point of the analysis is the extraordinary growth of public health and social medicine throughout Europe. Behind the process of the institutionalisation of hygiene and social medicine, we find a network of actors who played the role of a leading elite. This network was the driving force for the creation of national and international platforms of power and influence worldwide. Although there were many actors playing differing roles in different nations and moments, these actors mostly followed the leadership of the Rockefeller Foundation and the Health Organization of the League of Nations. Both organisations played a hegemonic role and infiltrated the national health authorities. They acted as political and financial powers, as a crystallisation nucleus for a new culture regarding contagious disease, expert training, and social hygiene policies. Under their influence a cohesive network of national experts in public health and political authorities gained considerable medico-political and technical power. This transnational force aimed to control, expand, and legitimise national and international initiatives in public health policies. Preventive medicine and public health was shaped as a professional field and a political issue by these powerful actors.

During the interwar years a surprisingly important event happened in most European nations: the spread of hygiene as a professional issue led to the establishment of national institutes of hygiene and national schools of public health. The institutionalisation of public health served as an instrument to establish research programmes around the new experimental medicine. The objective was to scientifically improve health standards, accelerate technical developments to fight disease, and implement national policies derived from transnational expertise and consensus. Consequently, biopolitics emerged as a powerful instrument of control and action against the social and demographic crises of the interwar years.

This powerful global phenomenon took place at a time when European countries were suffering the catastrophes of war, widespread urbanisation, migratory movements, deep social conflicts, financial crises, and huge epidemics.

The powerful emergence of experimental and social medicine in the political sphere can be seen as a stage in the evolution of the liberal state towards a *providential* or welfare state, an attempt to mitigate the negative consequences of capitalist expansion by means of liberal reformism. The new institutions associated with hygiene achieved an important political influence, when disease – individual and social – became a political issue. Moreover, hygiene institutes and schools of public health flourished at a time when bacteriology, serology, and experimental medicine opened huge expectations of success in the fight against epidemics, contagious diseases, and other social problems. The predominantly technical viewpoint understated the importance of poverty, exclusion, and social inequality as the chief pathogenic factors. Public health experts, serologists, and bacteriologists became powerful actors and these new professionals helped build a healthier society.

During the interwar years, *social hygiene* and *social medicine* were in the forefront of the international political agenda. National and international *biopolitics* launched a technical response to the health problems caused by poor living conditions and the social-economic crisis suffered in many European countries. However, experimental hygiene and social medicine strategies attempted to resolve socio-medical problems by combining social reformism and laboratory technology. The political and ideological influence of social hygiene opened a whole new medical field of research and intervention. Therefore, during the first half of the twentieth century we find an increased interest in health statistics and the prevention of disease and healthcare organisation. Most European countries experienced public and parliamentary debates on the collectivisation of healthcare and state intervention. Europe had become fertile ground for sanitary legislation, public health campaigns, the institutionalisation of public health, and public information on hygiene. Together with an increasing number of dispensaries, laboratories, institutes of health, and hospitals, these concerns and debates gave exceptional importance to the role of the public health expert.

Previous pages show how the strategies and arguments for the establishment of national institutes and schools of hygiene were similar in most European countries. They were supported by the need to fight epidemics and infectious diseases using new bacteriological and serological technologies. Furthermore, national institutions reinforced national identities and predicted improved health, modernity, and greater prosperity.

There was a common enemy: infectious disease and other health problems associated with social degeneration (including alcoholism, syphilis, tuberculosis, and mental disease). Poverty was in the background and experimental medicine was called on to complement or even supplement social reforms. These challenges to infectious disease became globalised due to the technocratic medical and social ideology spread by the hegemonic groups enjoying the financial support of the Rockefeller Foundation. The new experimental medicine relied on laboratory technologies: bacteriology, serology, vaccines, chemical and bacteriological treatment of water, food quality control, sewage systems, and disinfection. Programmes of social hygiene were supported by inspectors, experimental facilities, and administrative platforms.

National institutes, scientists, and research groups competed for prestige and international recognition. But despite rivalry and competition, the various organisations involved in the international and national networks during the interwar years sometimes appeared as a cohesive and dominant power. Nevertheless, their relations were also problematic on certain issues: provoking tensions, rivalry, and sometimes conflicts. There were debates regarding priorities and struggles between scientists and institutions. Indeed, international commissions were often forced to negotiate, but collaboration in the scientific domain usually prevailed. The collaborative forces that drove cohesion around common interests usually won the day. International standards had to be agreed on diagnoses of the causes of death and disease, doses of sera and vaccines, standards for biological products, hormones, and pharmaceuticals. Cooperation and competition between national and research groups were balanced. National institutes of hygiene represented an intermediate stage before the arrival of the unstoppable and almighty multinational health industry.

British, American, French, and German groups led most of the research lines, international research groups, and expert committees. Nevertheless, research programmes and groups often had a transnational dimension and were seldom reduced to a national issue. In some European countries, experimental public health was supported by the government as a part of the state administration. In other nations, the impulse came from university groups or private entities.

Should we conclude that the spread of national institutes of hygiene was simply the result of an evolving medical technology that had gained greater scientific and political influence and therapeutic efficiency? Was the spread of such institutes mainly the consequence of a process of imitation and rivalry among large research groups and institutions? The previous pages clearly show that this was not the case. Experimental medicine opened the possibility of focusing on social hygiene from a mostly technical perspective, and leaving the social causes of disease, poverty, and degeneration out of the debate. The nine departments of the Johns Hopkins School of Public Health showed the future of social medicine in the 1920s: public health administration; epidemiology; biometry and vital statistics; medical zoology; bacteriology; immunology; physiological hygiene; chemical hygiene; and filterable viruses. This pattern was sponsored and imitated internationally with little dissent. All the leading actors benefited from the model.

State public health programmes were predicated on the creation of professional elites of experts, who, building their expertise on statistical evidence, technical laboratory knowledge, and practical training in the field, served as authoritative referees for state policies, national and international campaigns, and the organisation of health services.

The huge amount of archival and printed sources discussed in the previous pages clearly shows that the globalisation of social medicine cannot be understood as a case of centre-periphery expansion, where prestigious and powerful nations and institutions influenced other peripheral countries. Neither was it a matter of appropriation of knowledge and technology. On the contrary: it was the consequence of an alliance between powerful experimental groups of experts from international organisations (League of Nations, International Labour Office, *Office Internationale d'Hygiène Publique*) and national authorities. Quietly pulling the strings in the background was the Rockefeller Foundation: which until the outbreak of World War Two, financed and carefully guided the development of national hygiene and public health in most countries. The foundation was the chief transnational motor of social medicine during the interwar years.

These actors, to a greater or lesser extent, contributed to the building of nations and the maintenance of public order. They also made scientific and technical contributions to national economies and competitiveness. This network of actors laid the foundations for the public health systems and globalised health industry that emerged after the end of World War Two.

Sources and bibliography

Sources

Balfour, A.; Porter, Ch. 'Public Health Training in the United States', Geneva: LONA, C.H.300, 1926.

Balfour, Public Health Training in the USA, Geneva: LONA, Doc. C.H.870, 1930.

Bayley, Ch. 'Public Health in Spain' 1926, Terrytown, New York: RAC, Record Group: 1.1. Projects, Series 795 Spain, folder 1.

Bernard, L. 'Public Health Training in Brazil, the Argentine and Uruguay', Geneva: LONA, C.H.866, 1926.

Bernard, L. 'Rapport sur l'enseignement de l'Hygiène en France', Geneva: LONA, C.H.134, 1923.

Bernard, L. 'Rapport sur cooperation avec les administrations sanitaires des Pays de l'Amerique Latine', Geneva: LONA, C.H.376, 8 October 1925.

Bernard, L. 'Committee on the Teaching of Hygiene. Report on the Teaching of Hygiene in Europe by . . .' Geneva: LONA, C.H.243, 1927.

Bernard, L. 'Report on the Conference held at the Inauguration of the Budapest and Zagreb Schools of Public Health', Geneva: LONA, C.H.661, 27 October, 1927.

Bernard, L. 'Report by Prof . . . on behalf of the Sub-Committee appointed to examine the French Government Proposal for the Creation of an International School of Advanced Health Studies at Paris', Terrytown, New York: RAC RG 6.1, series 1.1, box 38, folder 466, 1930.

'Bibliography of the technical work of the Health Organisation of the League of Nations, 1920–1945', *Quarterly Bulletin of the Health Organisation of the League of Nations*, 15, 1945, pp. 1–235.

Bourgeois, L. *Pour la Société des Nations*, Paris: E. Fasquelle, 1909.

Briand, A. 'Création à Paris, sous les auspices de la Société des Nations, d'un centre international de Hautes Études d'Hygiène', Geneva: LONA, C.538.1930.III.

Bucharest Institute of Sero-Therapeutics (1902–1923), Bucharest, 1923.

Buen, Sadí de; Luengo, E. 'Poder tripanolítico del suero de un enfermo tratado por el Bayer 205', *Archivos del Instituto Nacional de Higiene de Alfonso XIII*, 2, 1923, pp. 53–56.

Buen, Sadí de; Luengo, E. 'Ensayos terapéuticos con el "Bayer 205" en dos casos de tripanosomiasis humana', *Archivos del Instituto Nacional de Higiene de Alfonso XIII*, 2, 1923, pp. 85–96.

Buen, Sadí de. 'Note préliminaire sur l'épidemiologie de la fièvre recurrente espagnole', *Annales de Parasitologie Humaine et Comparée*, IV, 1926, pp. 185–192.

Carozzi, Dr. 'On the work of the Health Service of the International Labour Office', Geneva: LONA, C.H.86, 11 May, 1923.

Catálogo razonado de la colección de piezas anatómicas del Museo de Sanidad e Higiene Pública, Madrid: Instituto de Salud Carlos III, 2017.

Chodzko, W. 'Public Health Training in Denmark', Geneva: LONA, C.H.361, 1926.

Chodzko, W. 'Report on Public Health Training in Roumania, presented by . . .', Geneva: LONA, C.H.475, 2 June, 1926.

Chodzko, W. 'The Methods of Recruiting Students for Schools of Hygiene', Geneva: LONA, C.H.628, 1927.

Chodzko, W. 'The Programme of Courses at the Polish State School of Hygiene', Geneva: LONA, C.H.627, 1927.

Chodzko, W. 'Collaboration between the different Schools of Hygiene', Geneva: LONA, C.H.645, 1927.

Comisión Central de Trabajos Antipalúdicos. *Memoria de la campaña contra el paludismo (1925–1927)*, Madrid: Ministerio de la Gobernación, Dirección General de Sanidad, 1928.

Congrès International de Bienfaissance de Francfort sur-le-Mein, Brussels, 1858.

'Cooperation between philanthropic associations', Geneva: LONA, S12, dos 50430, 1926, 1 doc, cart 699.

'Cours internationale d'Hygiène' organisé par le Commité d'Hygiène de la Société des Nations à la Faculté de Médecine de Paris', Geneva: LONA, C.H./E.P.S./123, 1927.

'Création à Paris, sous les auspices de la Société des Nations, d'un Centre International de Hautes Études d'Hygiène', Geneva: LONA, C.535.1930.III, 1930.

'Création à Paris d'une École Internationale de Hautes Études d'Hygiène. Rapport du Comité d'Hygiène au Conseil de la Société des Nations relative à la proposition du gouvernement français', Geneva: LONA, C.589.1930.III, 1930.

'Creation of an Institute of Hygiene in Cuba', Geneva: LONA, dos. 54663, 1 doc., cart. 988, 1926.

Cumming, H.S. 'The Training of Sanitarians in the United States', Geneva: LONA, C.H.133, 1928.

Declaration of Human Rights, Geneva: United Nations, 1948.

'Décret Ministériel sur l'établissement et organisation de l'Institut Central d'Hygiène à Belgrade', Geneva: LONA, 1924.

'Enquiry into Public Health Administration and Health Insurance', Geneva: LONA, dos. 46868, 25 docs, cart. 968–972, 1925.

Escuela Nacional de Sanidad. Reglamento y Programas, Madrid: Imprenta José Molina, 1926.

'Exposición que precede al RD de 12 de abril de 1930, donde se establecen las justificaciones para la elaboración de un nuevo Reglamento de la Escuela Nacional de Sanidad', Madrid: *Gaceta*, 22 April 1930.

Fodéré, F.E. 'Lazaret'. In: *Dictionnaire Encyclopédique des Sciences Médicales*, Paris: G. Masson and P. Asselin, 1817.

Frank J.P. *De populorum miseria: morborum genitrice*, Ticini: Delectus Opusculorum Medicorum; 1790. vol. IX, pp. 302–324.

Frey, G. 'Die Organisation des Gesundheitswesens in Deutschen Verwaltungsgebiet von Russisch-Polen (Stand von 1 Oktober 1916)', *Zeitschrift fur Srztliche Fortbildung*, 5, 1917.

'Grant for the maintenance of a system of interchange of public health personnel on an international scale', Terrytown, New York, RAC, RG1.1. Series 100, Box 21, Folder 175, 1930.

'Health Centres in Yugoslavia', Geneva: LONA, dos. 55556, 1 doc., cart. 991, 1926.

History of the Norwegian Institute of Public Health. https://www.fhi.no/en/about/about-niph/this-is-the-norwegian-institute-of-public-health/history-of-the-norwegian-institute/ [Accessed 10th July, 2017].

Informe de la Comisión del Instituto Nacional de Higiene Alfonso XIII relativa a las posesiones españolas del Golfo de Guinea para el estudio de la enfermedad del sueño y de las condiciones sanitarias de la colonia... Dr. Gustavo Pittaluga, jefe de la comisión... Prólogo del director del Instituto D. Santiago Ramón y Cajal, Madrid: Ministerio de Estado, Sección Colonial, 1910.

'International Continuation Course in Public Health. London, 3 November–15 December 1927', Geneva: LONA, C.H./E.P.S./123, 1927.

'Institut d'Hygiène. Cours International d'Hygiène organisé sur l'initiative et avec le concours du Comité d'Hygiène de la Société des Nations. Université de Paris, Faculté de Médecine, année scolaire 1926–1927', Geneva: LONA, C.H./E.P.S./123, 1927.

'Institute of Hygiene [in Poland]', Terrytown, New York: RAC, IHB Minutes, 5 May 1922, RG 1.1. series 789, box 1, folder 1.

'Institute of Hygiene [in Poland]', Terrytown, New York: RAC, 23 May 1922, RG 1.1. series 789, box 1, folder 1.

Jitta, J. 'The Teaching of Hygiene in the Netherlands', Geneva: LONA, C.H.286, 3 April 1925.

Johan, B. 'The Training of Public Health Officers in Hungary', Geneva: LONA, C.H.630, 1927.

Johan, B. 'Relations between Hygienic Institutes in various countries and possible means of cooperation', Geneva: LONA, C.H.644, 1927.

Johan, B. 'Teaching public health in Hungary', Geneva: LONA, Doc. C.H.873 and 865, 1930.

Jorge, R. 'Public Health Training in the Netherlands', Geneva: LONA, Doc. C.H.389, 1926.

Kacprzak, M. 'The School of Public Health in Warsaw', Geneva: LONA, Doc. C.H.872.

Kaminski, Dr. The Health Organization of Roumania, Bucharest : 1923.

'Letter from W. Rose to L. Rajchman, 6 July 1922, Terrytown, New York, RAC, Archives of the Joint Distribution Committee, File 362.

Letter from L. Rajchman to Wickliffe Rose, Terrytown, New York: RAC RG 1.1, series 100, box 20, folder 165, 1922.

'Letter from L. Rajchman to C. Weynon, 9 April 1923', LONA, 12B 27967/26533, 1923.

'Letter from the Secretary-General of the League of Nations to the Foreign Office, 18 February, 1924 regarding the Establishment in London of a School of Hygiene'. LONA, 1213/34087, 1924.

'Letter from Selskar M. Gunn to Norman White on sanitary reforms in Hungary', Geneva: LONA, 1283/29308/26249, 19 November 1925.

'Letter from S. Gunn to F.F. Russell', Institute of Hygiene, 1922–1924, Terrytown, New York: RAC, series 789, box 1, folder 1, folder 1, 19 September 1924.

'Letter from S. Gunn to F.F. Russell', Institute of Hygiene, 1925–1929, Terrytown, New York: RAC, RF, series 789, box 1, folder 1–3, 13 April 1925.

'Letter from S. Gunn to F.F. Russell', Terrytown, New York: RAC, RG 1.1, series 100, box 20, folder 169, 23 October 1925.

'Letter from S. Deutschman to George K. Strode', Terrytown, New York: RAC, 6 April 1942, RG 1.1, series 100, box 22, folder 182, 1942–44.

Liebermann, I. L'Institut d'Hygiène de Budapest, Budapest, 1909.

'Liste des auditeurs du Cours International d'Hygiène organisé par l'Institut d'Hygiène de la Faculté de Médecine de Paris sur l'initiative et avec le concours du Comité d'Hygiène de la Société des Nations', Geneva, LONA, 13/1/1927, C.H./E.P.S./124, 1927.

Luengo, E. 'Nuevas investigaciones en un caso mortal de tripanosomiasis humana tratado por el Bayer 205'. *Archivos del Instituto Nacional de Higiene de Alfonso XIII*, 3, 1924, pp. 203–210.

'Memorandum on the Organization and functions of the Ministry of Health (England and Wales)'. Ministry of Health, March 1925, Geneva: LONA, 123/47764/26249, 1925.

Memoria de la Dirección General de Sanidad, Madrid: Ministerio de la Gobernación, 1943–1945.

Memoria de la Dirección General de Sanidad, Madrid: Ministerio de la Gobernación, 1948.

Ministerio de la Gobernación, Proyecto de un Instituto Nacional de Higiene (Bacteriología. Vacunación. Sueroterapia. Análisis química. Desinfección). Grases, arquitecto, Madrid: Imprenta Enrique Teodoro y Alonso, 1901.

Ministry of Public Health, Labour and Social Welfare. *General review of the health position in Roumania*, Bucharest: 1923.

Monin, E. Rapport sur l'Exposition d'Hygiène de Varsovie, Paris, Société des Nations, Organisation d'Hygiène, 1888.

'National Health Organisations: General', Geneva: LONA, series 23597, 1 dos., cart 6141, 1934.

'National Health Organisations: Countries', Geneva: LONA, series 1263, 38 dos., cart 6069, 1932–1946.

Newman, G. 'Health Education in Great Britain', Geneva: LONA, C.H.362, 1925.

Newman, G. 'On facilities available in England for the training of medical men for the Public Health Diploma', Geneva: LONA, dos. 2823, 1 doc, cart. 922, 1923.

Newman, G. 'Commission on Public Health Instruction. Meeting of October 6, 1925. Remarks of Sir . . .'. Geneva: LONA, C.H.375, 1925.

Nocht, B. 'Report on the academic teaching of Hygiene and social medicine at German universities, technical high schools and academies for social hygiene', Geneva: LONA, C.H.277, 17 March, 1925.

'Organisation and Administration of the Health Institute of Poland and of its School of Hygiene', Geneva: LONA, C.H. 414, 1925.

Onania, or the Heinous Sin of Self-Pollution, And All Its Frightful Consequences, in both Sexes, Considere'd with Spiritual and Physical Advice to Those, who have already injur'd themselves by this abominable practice ... London, H. Cooke, 1756.

Ortíz de Landazuri, A.; Luengo, E., 'Spain'. In: *International Health Year-Book 1924. Reports on the Public Health Progress of Twenty-Two Countries*, Geneva, League of Nations, 1925, pp. 361–402.

Ottolenghi, D. 'Public Health Training in the French and American Faculties of Medicine at Beirut', Geneva: LONA, Doc. C.H.410, 1926.

Ottolenghi, D., 'Public Health Training in Switzerland', Geneva: LONA, C.H.409, 1926.

París Eguilaz, H. Contribución al estudio de la epidemiología de la enfermedad del sueño en los territorios españoles del Golfo de Guinea. Trabajo dedicado al Comité Internacional de Higiene de la Sociedad de Naciones, Madrid: Espasa-Calpe, 1932.

Pelc, H. 'Preliminary Report on Programmes of Schools of Public Health', Geneva: LONA, C.H.623, 1927.

Pelc, H. 'Supplementary Report on Programmes of Schools of Public Health', Geneva: LONA, C.H.623 (a), 1927.

Pittaluga, G. 'Noticia sobre la Tripanosomiasis humana (enfermedad del sueño) en las posesiones españolas del Golfo de Guinea', *Boletín del Instituto de Sueroterapia, Vacunación y Bacteriología de Alfonso XIII*, 5, 1909, pp. 135–141.

Pittaluga, G. La tripanosomiasis humana (enfermedad del sueño) en las posesiones españolas del Golfo de Guinea. Primer informe del Dr... Jefe de la Comisión del Instituto de Alfonso XIII enviada por el Ministerio de Estado a dichas Posesiones. Mayo-Noviembre, 1909, Madrid: Instituto Nacional de Higiene de Alfonso XIII, Imprenta y Librería de Nicolás Moya, 1910.

Pittaluga, G. *La constitución de la Escuela Nacional de Sanidad*, Madrid: Publicaciones de la Escuela Nacional de Sanidad, 1930.

Pittaluga, G.; De Buen, S.; Benzo. M. 'Organismos centrales de investigación y enseñanza sanitarias y sus relaciones con los demás Centros sanitarios'. In: Nájera, L. (ed.) *Primer Congreso Nacional de Sanidad*, Madrid: Ministerio de la Gobernación, 1934, 5–15.

Prausnitz, C. 'Report on teaching public health in Europe', Geneva: LONA, Doc. C.H.873 and 865, 1930.

'Proposed collective studies of specific public health problems', Geneva: LONA, dos. 33803, 1 doc, cart. 923, 1924.

'Provisional Programme of Courses for (Medical) candidates for positions in the Hungarian Public Health Service', Geneva: LONA, 1927.

'Public Health Instruction: General', Geneva: LONA, series 879, 1 dos., cart 6089, 1932–1933.

'Public Health and Medical Services', Geneva, LONA, Series 21641, 5 dos., cart 6141, 1935–1944.

Rajchman, L.W. *The League of Nations Health Organisation: What it is and how it works?* Terrytown, New York: RAC, 18 November 1921, RG 1.1, Series 100, Box 20, Folder 165.

Rajchman, L.W. 'Report on the Epidemic Situation in Eastern Europe', RAC, RG 1.1, Series 100, Box 20, Folder 165, 18 February 1922.

Rajchman, L.W. Review of the Experience, 1927.

Rajchman, L.W. 'Instruction to all the States, 14.01.1925 by Rajchman', Geneva: LONA, 12B/42592/41461/Box R953/1919–1927.

Rapport Épidémiologique Annuel, Genève: Société des Nations, 1923.

'Report on the Work of the First Session, February 11th to 21st, 1924', Geneva: LONA, Health Committee, League of Nations, C.63.1924 [C.H.192.], 22 February, 1924.

'Report of the Health Committee to the Permanent Committee...', Geneva: LONA, A.22.1924.III.

'Report on the Conference on Schools of Public Health held at Budapest and Zagreb from September 29th to October 4th, 1927', Geneva, LONA, C.H.659, 1927.

'Reports on Schools of Public Health', Geneva: LONA, Doc. C.H.873 and 865, 1927.

'Resumen de la labor realizada por la Escuela Nacional de Sanidad durante el cuso 1931–1932', *Revista de Sanidad e Higiene Pública*, 8:1, 1933, pp. 66–70.

Rockefeller Foundation, The: A Digital History. Essays, biographies and thousands of digitalized documents. Https://rockfound.rockarch.org.

Rose, W. 'Epidemic control in Europe, and the League.' *American Review of Reviews*, 46, 1922, p. 2.

Rosen, G. 'Economic and Social Policy in the Development of Public Health. An Essay in Interpretation.' *Journal of the History of Medicine and Allied Sciences*, 8, 1953, pp. 406–430.

Rosen G. 'Cameralism and the Concept of Medical Police'. *Bulletin of the History and Medicine*, 27, 1953, pp. 21–42.

Rosen, G. 'The Fate of the Concept of Medical Police'. *Centaurus*, 5, 1957, pp. 97–113.

Rosen, G. 'Mercantilism and Health Policy in Eighteenth Century French Thought'. *Medical History*, 3, 1959, pp. 259–277.

Ruiz–Falcó, F., 'Escuela Nacional de Sanidad. Problemática pasada, actual y futura'. *Revista de Sanidad e Higiene Pública*, 57, 1983, pp. 359–372.

Ruíz-Falcó, F. 'Mis recuerdos en la Escuela Nacional de Sanidad'. In *Homenaje a la Escuela Nacional de Sanidad con motivo de su 70 aniversario*, Madrid: 1994.

Salomonsen, C.J. (ed.) Contributions from the University Laboratory for Medical Bacteriology, to celebrate the inauguration of the State Serum Institute, Copenhagen, O.C. Olsen & Co., 1902.

San Martín, A. *La Conferencia Sanitaria Internacional de Dresde*, Madrid, Imprenta de Ricardo Rojas, 1883.

'School Hygiene Interchange', Geneva: LONA, dos. 29549, 1923, 12 docs, cart 900–901, 1924.

Serret, R. 'La vacuna en el extranjero'. Boletín del Instituto de Sueroterapia, Vacunación y Bacteriología de Alfonso XIII, 2, 1906, pp. 177–182.

Sigerist, H.E. 'From Bismarck to Beveridge. Developments and Trends in Social Security Legislation'. *Bulletin of the History of Medicine*, 13, 1943, pp. 365–388.

Société des Nations, Genève: Société des Nations, 1931, p. 18.

Stampar, A. 'The Zagreb School of Hygiene', Geneva: LONA, C.H.417, 1927.

Stampar, A. 'Supplementary note relating to training at the School of Hygiene, at Zagreb.' Geneva: LONA, C.H.417 (a), 1927.

Stampar, A. 'The School of Public Health in Zagreb', Geneva: LONA, Doc. C.H.873 and 865, 1930.

Swellengrebel, N.H. *Informe sobre el viaje a España.* Boletín Técnico de la Dirección General de Sanidad. Marzo, 1926, Madrid: Comité de Paludismo, Ministerio de la Gobernación, Dirección General de Sanidad, 1927.

Tello, F.; Ruiz Falcó, A. 'La peste bubónica en la zona de influencia española en Marruecos'. *Boletín del Instituto de Sueroterapia, Vacunación y Bacteriología de Alfonso XIII*, 10, 1914, pp. 97–143.

Ten Years of World Co-operation . . . Secretariat of the League of Nations in Geneva, London: Hazell, Watson & Viney, 1930.

'The Royal Institute of Public Health', Geneva: LONA, 8480.

The School of Hygiene and Public Health of the Johns Hopkins University, Baltimore: The American Journal of Hygiene Monographic Series, 1926.

'The State Hygienic Institute, Prague, Czechoslovakia. Outline of the working program of the Institute', Geneva: LON Archives, 1925.

Tissot, S.A. *L'Onanisme: Dissertation sur les Maladies produites para la Masturbation*, Laussanne: Chez Marc Chapuis et Cie, 1761.

'United States Public Health Service reports', Geneva: LONA, dos. 41628, 1 doc., cart. 954, 1925.

Vacek, B.; Pelc, H., 'Report on teaching public health in Prague', Geneva: LONA, doc. C.H.871, 1930.

Vingt-cinq ans d'activité de l'Office International d'Hygiène Publique, 1909–1933, Paris, OIHP, 1933.

Zinsser, H. 'Report on Journey to Russia as Epidemic Commissioner of Hygienic Section, League of Nations, from June 11th to July 20th, 1923', Terrytown, New York: RAC, RG 1.1, Series 100, Box 22, Folder 183. [Published at the League of Nations Health Section, Reports 1922–1925].

Bibliography

Ackerknecht, E.H. 'Anticontagionism between 1821 and 1867'. *Bulletin of the History of Medicine*, 22, 1948, pp. 562–593.

Ackerknecht, E.H. *A Short History of Medicine*, Baltimore: Johns Hopkins University Press, 1982.

Aldous, Ch.; Suzuki, A. *Reforming Public Health in Occupied Japan, 1945–52 Alien prescriptions?* London & New York: Routledge, 2012.

Amrith, S.S. *Decolonizing International Health, India and South Asia, 1930–1965*, Hampshire: Palgrave, 2006.

Anderson, W. 'Postcolonial Histories of Medicine.' In F. Huisman and J. Harley (eds). *Locating Medical History: The Stories and their Meanings*. Baltimore: Johns Hopkins University Press, 2004, pp. 285–306.

Anderson, W. 'Making Global Health History: The Postcolonial Worldliness of Biomedicine', *Social History of Medicine*, 27, 2014, pp. 372–384.

Andresen, A.; Barona, J.L.; Cherry, S. (eds), *Making a New Countryside? Health Policies and Practices in European History c. 1860–1950*, Frankfurt am Main: PIE Peter Lang, 2010.

Andresen, A.; Hubbard, W.; Ryymin, T. (eds) *International and Local Approaches to Health and Health Care*, Oslo: Novus Press, 2010.

Andresen, A.; Gronlie, T.; Hubbard, W.; Ryymin, T. (eds) *Health Care Systems and Medical Institutions*, Oslo: Novus Press, 2009.

Argote, L.; Ingram, P. 'Knowledge Transfer: A Basis for Competitive Advantage in Firms'. In *Organizational Behavior and Human Decision Processes*, 82, 2000, pp. 150–169.

Armitage, D. *Foundations of Modern International Thought*, Cambridge: Cambridge University Press, 2013.

Arnold, D. *Colonizing the Body. State Medicine and Epidemic Disease in Nineteenth-Century India*, Berkeley: The University of California Press, 1993.

Ashford, D. *The Emergence of the Welfare States*, Oxford: Blackwell, 1986.

Ashford, D. 'Intergovernmental social transfers and the welfare state', *Government and Policy*, 8, 1990, pp. 217–232.

Azuma, E. *Between Two Empires: Race, History, and Transnationalism in Japanese America*, New York: Oxford University Press, 2005.

Baily, Ch. A. et al.: 'AHR Conversation: On Transnational History', *American Historical Review*, 111, 2006, pp. 1441–1464.

Baldwin, P. *Contagion and the State in Europe 1830–1930*, Cambridge: Cambridge University Press, 1999.

Balinska, M.A. *Une vie pour l'humanitaire: Ludwik Rajchman 1881–1965*, Paris, La Découverte, 1995.

Balinska, M.A. 'Assistance and Not Mere Relief: the Epidemic Commission of the League of Nations', in Weindling P. (ed.), *International Health Organisations and Movements 1918–1939*. Cambridge, Cambridge University Press, 1995, pp. 81–108.

Balinska, M.A. 'The National Institute of Hygiene and Public Health in Poland 1918–1939'. *Social History of Medicine*, 9, 1996, pp. 427–445.

Barbalet, J. *Citizenship*, Milton Keynes: Open University Press, 1988.

Barnes, D.S. The Great Stink of Paris and the Nineteenth-Century Struggle against Filth and Germs, Baltimore: The Johns Hopkins University Press, 2006.

Barona Vilar, J.L. *The Rockefeller Foundation, Public Health and International Diplomacy*, London: Pickering and Chatto, 2015.

Barona Vilar, J.L. *Food Inspection in Denmark. Reports on meat and milk presented to the League of Nations on the occasion of the visit of European Health Officers in 1924*, Estrup: Danish Agricultural Museum, 2015.

Barona Vilar, J.L. *La medicalización del hambre. Economía política de la alimentación en Europa*, Barcelona: Icaria, 2014.

Barona Vilar, J.L. *The Problem of Nutrition: Experimental Science, Public Health and Economy in Europe 1914–1945*, Brussels: Peter Lang, 2010.

Barona, Vilar J.L. (ed.) *El exilio científico republicano*, Valencia: PUV, 2010.

Barona Vilar, J.L. *From Hunger to Malnutrition: The Political Economy of Scientific Knowledge in Europe, 1918–1960*, Frankfurt am Main: Peter Lang, 2012.

Barona Vilar, J.L. 'In the Name of Health. The *Instituto Nacional de Higiene Alfonso XIII* and laboratory campaigns in Spanish rural áreas and African colonies, 1910–1924'. In Andresen, A.; Gronlie, T.; Hubbard, W.; Ryymin, T. (eds) *Health Care Systems and Medical Institutions*, Oslo: Novus Press, 2009, pp. 154–169.

Barona Vilar, J.L. 'Public Health Experts and Scientific Authority'. In Andresen, A.; Hubbard, W.; Ryymin, T. (eds.) *International and Local Approaches to Health and Health Care*, Oslo: Novus Press, 2010, pp. 31–48.

Barona Vilar, J.L.; Bernabeu-Mestre, J. *La Salud y el Estado. El movimiento sanitario internacional y la administración española (1851–1945)*, Valencia: Publicaciones de la Universidad de Valencia, 2008.

Barona Vilar, J.L.; Cherry, S. (eds.) *Health and Medicine in Rural Europe (1850–1945)*, Valencia: Publicaciones de la Universidad de Valencia/Seminari d'Estudis sobre la Ciència, 2005.

Barona Vilar, J.L., Micó, J (eds) *Salut i Malaltia en els Municipis Valencians*, Valencia: Seminari d'Estudis sobre la Ciència, 1996.

Basalla, G. 'The Spread of Western Science', *Science*, 156, 1967, pp. 111–122.

Bedetti, C.; De Castro, P.; Modigliani, S. *Atti del Convegno Storie e memorie dell'Istituto Superiore di Sanità*, Roma: Istituto Superiore di Sanità, 2008.

Ben-David, J. *The Scientist's Role in Society: A Comparative Study*, Chicago: University of Chicago Press, 1971.

Ben-David, J. *Centres of Learning: Britain, France, Germany, United States (Foundations of Higher Education) by Carnegie Commission on Higher Education*, New York: Piscataway-MacGraw-Hill, 1977.

Ben-David, J. *Scientific Growth: Essays on the Social Organization and Ethos of Science (California Studies in the History of Science)*. Edited by Gad Freudenthal, Berkeley: University of California Press, 1991.

Bender, Th. (ed.) *Rethinking American History in a Global Age*, Berkeley: University of California Press, 2002.

Bender, Th. *A Nation Among Nations: America's Place in World History*, New York: Hill and Wang, 2006.

Berliner, H.S. *A System of Scientific Medicine: Philanthropic Foundations in the Flexner Era*, New York and London: Tavistock, 1985.

Bernabeu-Mestre, Josep, 'La utopía reformadora de la Segunda República: la labor de Marcelino Pascua al frente de la Dirección General de Sanidad, 1931–1933', *Revista Española de Salud Pública*, 74, 2000, pp. 1–13.

Bernabeu-Mestre, J. *La salud pública que no va poder ser. José Estellés Salarich (1896–1990): una aportació valenciana a la sanitat espanyola contemporània*, València: Consell Valencià de Cultura (Serie Minor, 62), 2007.

Beveridge, W. *Social Insurance and Allied Services*, London: HMSO, 1942.

Beveridge, W. *Voluntary Action*, London: Allen and Unwin, 1948.

Bhattacharya, S. 'Global and Local Histories of Medicine: Interpretative Challenges and Future Possibilities'. In *The Oxford Handbook of the History of Medicine*. Jackson, M. (ed.), Oxford: Oxford University Press, 2011, pp. 135–149

Bhattacharya, S. 'The World Health Organization and Global Smallpox Eradication', *Journal of Epidemiology and Community Health*, 62 (10), 2008, pp. 909–912.

Birn, A.E. 'A Global Perspective: Reframing the History of Health, Medicine, and Disease', *Global Public Health*, 4, 2009, pp. 50–68.

Birn, A.E.; Pillay, Y.; and Holtz, T.H., *Textbook of Global Health*, 4th edition, Oxford: Oxford University Press, 2017.

Birn, A.E.; Brown, Th. (eds) *Comrades in Health: US Health Internationalists, Abroad and at Home*, New Brunswick, Rutgers University Press, 2013.

Blümel, P.; Gerber, K.; Timm, H., *100 Jahre Robert Koch-Institut*, Berlin: Robert Koch-Institut, 1991.

Bulmer, M. 'Edward Shils, as a Sociologist', *Minerva*, 34, (1), 1996, pp. 7–21.

Boiling, L.R.; Smith, C. *Private Foreign Aid: US Philanthropy for Relief and Development*, Boulder, CO: Westview Press, 1982.

Bonastra Tolós, J. *Ciencia, sociedad y planificación territorial en la institución del lazareto*, Barcelona, Tesis Doctoral, Publicacions de la Universitat de Barcelona, 2006.

Borowy, I. *Coming to Terms with World Health: The League of Nations Health Organisation 1921–1946*, Frankfurt am Main: Peter Lang, 2009.

Borowy, I. 'World Health in a Book – The International Health Yearbooks'. In I. Borowy and W.D. Gruner (eds.) *Facing Illness in Troubled Times: Health in Europe in the Interwar Years 1918–1939*, Frankfurt am Main: PIE Peter Lang, 2005, pp. 85–128.

Borowy, I.; Gruner, W.D. (eds) *Facing Illness in Troubled Times: Health in Europe in the Interwar Years 1918–1939*, Frankfurt am Main: PIE Peter Lang, 2005.

Boyce, R. *The Great Interwar Crisis and the Collapse of Globalisation*, Hampshire: Palgrave MacMillan, 2012.

Brandt, A.M.; Gardner, M. 'Antagonism and Accommodation: Interpreting the Relationship between Public Health and Medicine in the United States during the 20th Century', *American Journal of Public Health*, 90, 2000, pp. 707–715.

Bremner, R.H. *American Philanthropy*, Chicago: University of Chicago Press, 1988.

Breschi, M.; Pozzi, L. (eds) *The Determinants of Infant and Child Mortality in Past European Populations*, Udine: Società Italiana di Demografia Storica, 2004.

Brock, ThD. *Robert Koch. A Life in Medicine and Bacteriology*, Berlin: Springer Verlag, 1988.

Brown, E.R. 'Public health and imperialism: Early Rockefeller programs at home and abroad', *American Journal of Public health*, 66, 1976, pp. 897–903.

Brown, E.R. *Rockefeller Medicine Men: Medicine and Capitalism in America*, Berkeley: University of California Press, 1979.

Brown, T.M.; Fee, E. 'Social Movements in Health', *Annual Review of Public Health*, 35, 2014, pp. 385–398.

Budde, G.; Conrad, S.; Janz, O. (eds) *Transnationale Geschichte: Themen, Tendenzen und Theorien*, Göttingen: Vandenhoeck & Ruprecht, 2006.

Bulmer, M. 'Edward Shils, as a sociologist', *Minerva*, 34 (1), 1996, pp. 7–21.

Canguilhem, G. *Le Normal et le Pathologique*, Paris: PUF, 1966.

Carnino, G. 'Louis Pasteur: Pure science serving industry', *Mouvement Sociale*, 248, 2014, pp. 9–28.

Cohn, B. *Colonialism and its Forms of Knowledge: The British in India*, Princeton: Princeton University Press, 1996.

Cook, G.C. *From the Greenwich Hulks to Old St. Pancras: A History of Tropical Disease in London*, London: Bloomsbury Academic Collections, 2015.

Cornebise, A. *Typhus and Doughboys, the American-Polish Typhus Relief Expedition 1919–21*, Delaware: University of Delaware Press, 1982.

Craig, G.A. 'The Historian and the Study of International Relations', *American Historical Review*, 88, 1983, pp. 1–11.

Cueto, M. (ed.) *Missionaries of Science: The Rockefeller Foundation and Latin America*, Bloomington: Indiana University Press, 1994.

Culpitt, I. *Welfare and Citizenship: Beyond the Crisis of the Welfare State?* London: Sage, 1992.

Curti, M. *American Philanthropy Abroad*, New Brunswick: Rutgers University Press, 1963.

Deacon, B. *Global Social Policy*, London: Sage, 1997.

Dean, H. *Welfare, Law and Citizenship*, Hemel Hempstead: Prentice Hall/ Harvester Wheatsheaf, 1996.

Debré, P. *Louis Pasteur*, Baltimore: Johns Hopkins University Press, 1998.

Dubin, M.D. 'The League of Nations and the Development of the Public Health Profession', Warwick, British International Studies Association, 1991.

Dugac, Z. 'Like Yeast in Fermentation: Public Health in Interwar Yugoslavia'. In: Promitzer, Ch.; Trubeta, S.; Turda, M. *Health, Hygiene and Eugenics in Southeastern Europe to 1945*, Budapest: Central University Press, 2011.

Elias, N. *Über den Prozeß der Zivilisation. Soziogenetische und psychogenetische Untersuchungen. Erster Band. Wandlungen des Verhaltens in den weltlichen Oberschichten des Abendlandes und Zweiter Band. Wandlungen der Gesellschaft. Entwurf einer Theorie der Zivilisation*, Basel: Verlag Haus zum Falken, 1939.

Elvbakken, K.T.; Ludvigsen, K. 'Medical Professional Practices, University Disciplines and the State: A Case Study from Norwegian Hygiene and Psychiatry 1800–1940', *Hygiea Internationalis*, 12 (2), 2016, pp. 7–28.

Evans, H. 'European Malaria Policy in the 1920s and 1930s: The Epidemiology of Minutiae', *Isis*, 80, 1989, pp. 45–49.

Farley, J. *To Cast Out Disease: A History of the International Health Division of the Rockefeller Foundation (1913–1951)*, Oxford: Oxford University Press, 2004.

Flora, P. (ed.) *State Formation, Nation-building and Mass Politics in Europe: The Theory of Stein Rokkan*, Oxford: Oxford University Press, 1996.

Foucault, M. *Il Faut Défendre la Société*, Paris: Éditions du Seuil, 1997.

Friedman, L.J.; McGarvie, M.D. (eds) *Charity, Philanthropy, and Civility in American History*, Cambridge: Cambridge University Press, 2003.

Geison, G.L. *The Private Science of Louis Pasteur*, Princeton: Princeton University Press, 1995.

Gesundheit schützen, Risiken erforschen. Wer wir sind, Worauf wir zurückblicken, Was wir leisten, Berlin: Robert Koch-Institut, 2011.

Geyer, M.H.; Paulmann, J. (eds.) *The Mechanics of Internationalism: Culture, Society, and Politics from the 1840s to the First World War*, Oxford: Oxford University Press, 2001.

Gibbons, M. et al. *The New Production of Knowledge: The Dynamics of Science and Research in Contemporary Societies*, London: Sage, 1994.

Gradmann, Ch. 'Money and Microbes: Robert Koch, Tuberculin and the Foundation of the Institute for Infectious Diseases in Berlin in 1891', *History and Philosophy of the Life Sciences*, 22, 2000, pp. 51–71.

Gradmann, Ch. *Krankheit im Labor: Robert Koch und die medizinische Bakteriologie*, Göttingen: Wallstein, 2005.

Gramsci, A. *Quaderni del carcere*, Roma: Einaudi, 1975.

Habermas, J. *The Crisis of the European Union: A Response*, Malden, MA: Polity Press, 2012.

Harris, S.J. 'Networks of Travel, Correspondence, and Exchange', in: *The Cambridge History of Science*, Cambridge University Press, 2006, vol 3, pp. 341–363.

Harrison, M. *Contagion. How commerce has spread disease*, Yale: Yale University Press, 2013.

Harrison, M. 'Disease, Diplomacy and International Commerce: The Origins of International Sanitary Regulation in the Nineteenth Century', *Journal of Global History*, 1, 2006, pp. 197–217.

Harrison, M. 'A Global Perspective: Reframing the History of Health, Medicine, and Disease', *Bulletin of the History of Medicine*, 89 (4), 2015, pp. 639–689.

Heater, D. *Citizenship*, Harlow: Longman, 1990.

Henig, R. *The League of Nations*, London: Haus Publishing, 2010.

Hewitt, M.; Powell, M. 'A different back to Beveridge?' In E. Brunsdon et al. (eds) *Social Policy Review*, 10, London: Social Policy Association, 1998.

Hill, D.M. *Citizens and Cities*, Hemel Hempstead: Harvester Wheatsheaf, 1994.

History of the Norwegian Institute of Public Health. See: https://www.fhi.no/en/about/ about-niph/this-is-the-norwegian-institute-of-public-health/history-of-the-norwegian-institute-/ [Accessed 10 July 2017].

Housden, M. *The League of Nations and the Organization of Peace*, New York: Pearson Longman, 2012.

Hodges, S. 'The Global Menace', *Social History of Medicine*, 25 (3), 2012, pp. 719–728.

Howard-Jones, N. 'International Public Health between the Two World Wars: The Organizational Problems', Geneva: World Health Organization, 1978.

Hubbard, W.H. 'Essay Review. Public Health in Norway 1603–2003', *Medical History*, 50, 2006, pp. 113–117.

Huisman, F.; Harley, J. (ed.) *Locating Medical History: The Stories and their Meanings*, Baltimore: Johns Hopkins University Press, 2004.

Hulverscheidt, M; Laukötter, A. (eds) *Infektion und Institution. Zur Wissenschaftgeschichte des Robert Koch-Institus im Nazionalsozialismus*, Göttingen: Wallstein Verlag, 2009.

Hüntelmann, A.C. 'Staatliche und kommunale Gesundheitspflege vor und nach dem Ersten Weltkrieg'. In Hofmann, W. (ed) *Fürsorge in Brandenburg: Entwicklungen, Kontinuitäten, Umbrüche*, Berlin: Be.Bra Wissenschaft Verlag, 2007.

Hüntelmann, A.C.; Vossen, J.; Czech, H. (ed.) *Gesundheit und Staat: Studien zur Geschichte der Gesundheitsämter in Deutschland, 1870–1950*, Husum: Matthiesen, 2006.

Hüntelmann, A.C. 'Diphtheriaserum and Serumtherapy – Development, Production and Regulation in fin de siècle Germany', *Dynamis*, 27, 2007, pp. 107–131.

Hüntelmann, A.C. *Hygiene im Namen des Staates*, Göttingen: Wallstein Verlag, 2008.

Hüntelmann, A.C. *Paul Ehrlich: Leben, Forschung, Ökonomien, Netzwerke*, Göttingen: Wallstein Verlag, 2012.

Hutchinson, J.F. *Champions of Charity: War and the Rise of the Red Cross*, Boulder, CO: Westview Press, 1996.

Inkster, I. 'Scientific Enterprise and the Colonial "Model": Observations on Australian Experience in Historical Context', *Social Studies of Science*, 15 (4), 1985, pp. 677–704.

Iriye, A. 'The Internationalization of History', *American Historical Review*, 94 (1), 1989, pp. 1–10.

Iriye, A.; Saunier, P.Y. (ed.) *The Palgrave Dictionary of Transnational History*, Basingstoke: Palgrave MacMillan, 2009.

Iriye, A. *Global and Transnational History: The Past, Present and Future*, Basingstoke: Palgrave MacMillan, 2013.

Johnson, R. 'Colonial Mission and Imperial Tropical Medicine: Livingston College, London, 1893–1914', *Social History of Medicine*, 23 (3), 2010, pp. 549–566.

Labisch, A. *Homo Hygienicus. Gesundheit und Medizin in der Neuzeit*, Frankfurt am Main: Campus, 1992.

Landrum, R.B.; Smith, C. *Private Foreign Aid: US Philanthropy for Relief and Development*, Boulder, CO: Westview Press, 1982.

Latour, B. *The Pasteurization of France*, Cambridge, MA: Harvard University Press, 1988.

Latour, B. *Reassembling the Social: An introduction to actor-network-theory*, Oxford: Oxford University Press, 2005.

Latour, B. *Science in Action: How to Follow Scientists and Engineers through Society*, Cambridge, MA: Harvard University Press, 1987.

League of Nations 1920–1946: Organization and Accomplishments. A Retrospective of the First Organization for the Establishment of World Peace, Geneva: United Nations, 1996.

Levitas, R. *The Inclusive Society?* Basingstoke: Macmillan, 1998.

Lipphardt, V.; Ludwig, D. 'Knowledge Transfer and Science Transfer', European History Online (EGO), Mainz: Institute of European History, 2011. See: http://www.ieg-ego.eu/lipphardtv- ludwigd-2011 [Accessed 20 July 2017].

Lister, R. *The Exclusive Society. Citizenship and the Poor*, London: CPAG, 1990.

Livingstone, D.N. *Putting Science in its Place: Geographies of scientific knowledge*, Chicago: University of Chicago Press, 2003.

Livingstone, D.N. 'Changing Climate, Human Evolution, and the Revival of Environmental Determinism', *Bulletin of the History of Medicine*, 86, 2012, pp. 564–595.

López Piñero, J.M. *Mateo Seoane, la introducción en España del sistema sanitario liberal, 1791–1870*, Madrid: Ministerio de Sanidad, 1984.

Löwy, I.; Zylberman, P. 'Introduction: Medicine as a Social Instrument: Rockefeller Foundation, 1913–45', *Studies in the History and Philosophy of Biology and Biomedical Sciences*, 31 (3), 2000, pp. 365–379.

MacLeod, R. 'On Visiting the "Moving Metropolis": Reflections on the Architecture of Imperial Science', *Historical Records of Australian Science*, 5, 1980, pp. 1–16.

MacLeod, R. (ed.) *Nature and Empire: Science and the Colonial Enterprise*, Chicago: Osiris, volume 15, 2000.

Marbeau, M. *La Société des Nations*, Paris: PUF, 2001.

Marchand, M.H. *Une Histoire de l'Institut Pasteur au coeur de la Santé Publique Mondiale*, Paris: Privat, 2015.

Marks, S. 'What is Colonial about Colonial Medicine? And what has happened to Imperialism and Health?', *Social History of Medicine*, 1, 1997, pp. 205–219.

Marshall, T.H. *Sociology at the Crossroads*, London: Heinemann, 1963.

Marshall, T.H. *Social Policy*, London: Hutchinson, 1970.

Marshall, T.H. *The Right to Welfare*, London: Heinemann,1981.

Másová, H. 'Social Hygiene and Social Medicine in Interwar Czechoslovakia with the 13th District of the City of Prague as its Laboratory', *Hygiea Internationalis: An Interdisciplinary Journal for the History of Public Health*, 6 (2), 2007, pp. 53–68.

McClellan, J.; Regourd, F. *The Colonial Machine: French Science and Overseas Expansion in the Old Regime*, Turnhout: Brepols, 2011.

Medina, R. 'Extracting the Spanish nation from Equatorial Guinea: Scientific technologies of national identity as colonial legacies', *Social Studies of Science*, 39, 2009, pp. 81–112.

Moran, M. 'The frontiers of social citizenship: the case of health care entitlements'. In Vogel, U.; Moran, M. (eds) *The Frontiers of Citizenship*, Basingstoke: Macmillan, 1991, pp. 32–57.

Morange, M. (org) *L'Institut Pasteur: Contributions à son histoire*, Paris: La Découverte, 1991.

Moseng, O.G. *Det offentilige helsevesen i Norge 1603–2003. Vol I: Ansvaret for undersattenes helse 1603–1850*, Oslo: Universiteitsforlaget, 2003.

Nájera Morrondo, R. 'El Instituto de Salud Carlos III y la sanidad española. Origen de la medicina de laboratorio, de los institutos de salud pública y de la investigación sanitaria', *Revista Española de Salud Pública*, 80, 2006, pp. 585–604.

Navarro García, R. *Historia de las Instituciones Sanitarias Nacionales*, Madrid: Instituto de Salud Carlos III, 2001.

Northedge, F.S. *The League of Nations: Its Life and Times, 1920–1946*, New York: Holmes & Meier, 1986.

Nowotny, H.; Scott, P.; Gibbons, M. *Re-Thinking Science. Knowledge and the Public in an Age of Uncertainty*, Cambridge, MA: Polity Press, 2001.

Ngai, M.M. 'Promises and Perils of Transnational History', *Perspectives on History*, December, 2012. See www.historians.org/publications-and-directories/perspectives-on-history/december-2012/the-future-of-the-discipline/promises-and-perils-of-transnational-history [Accessed, 16 June 2017].

Nye, J.S.; Keohane, R. 'Transnational Relations and World Politics', *International Organization*, 25 (3), 1971, pp. 329–349.

Oosterhuis, H. *Health and Citizenship. Political Cultures of Health in Modern Europe*, London and New York: Routledge, 2016.

Packard, R.M. *A History of Global Health: Interventions into the Lives of Other Peoples*, Baltimore: Johns Hopkins University Press, 2016.

Page, B.B.; Valone, D.A. (eds) *Philanthropic Foundations and the Globalization of Scientific Medicine and Public Health*, Lanham: University Press of America, 2007.

Paillette, C. 'Épidémies, Santé et Ordre Mondial. Le Rôle des Organisations Sanitaires Internationales, 1903–1923', *Monde(s): Histoire, Espaces, Relations*, 2 (2), 2012, pp. 235–256.

Palladino, P.; Worboys, M. 'Science and Imperialism', *Isis*, 84 (1), 1993, pp. 91–102.

Palladino, P. 'Historical Perspectives on Science, Society and the Political'. In Pestre, D. (ed.) *Report to the Science, Economy and Society Directorate*, Bruxelles, European Commission, 2007, pp. 105–107.

Palmer, S. *Launching Global Health: The Caribbean Odyssey of the Rockefeller Foundation*, Michigan: University of Michigan Press, 2010.

Parnas, J. 'Throvald Madsen 1870–1957. Leader in international public health', *Danish Medical Bulletin*, 28, 1981, pp. 82–86.

Patel, K.K. *Nach der Nationalfixiertheit: Perspektiven einer transnationalen Geschichte*, Berlin: Öffentliche Vorlesungen der Humboldt-Universität zu Berlin, 2004.

Patel, K.K. 'Transnational History', *European History online, 2010-12-03*. See: http://ieg-ego.eu/en/threads/theories-and-methods/transnational-history [Accessed 6 April 2017].

Petersen, K.; Stewart, J.; Sørensen, M.K. (eds) *American Foundations and the European Welfare States*, Odense: University of Odense, 2013.

Petitjean, P.; Jami, C.; Moulin, A.M. (eds) *Science and Empires: Historical Studies about Scientific Development and European Expansion*, Boston: Springer Boston Studies in the History of Science, 1992.

Pons, J.; Rodríguez, S. (eds) Los orígenes del Estado del Bienestar en España, 1900–1945. Los seguros de accidentes, vejez, desempleo y enfermedad, Zaragoza: Prensas Universitarias, 2011.

Porter, D. *Health, Civilisation and the State: A History of Public Health from Antiquity to Modernity*, Abingdon, Routledge, 1999.

Porras Gallo, M.I. 'Antecedentes y creación del Instituto de Sueroterapia, Vacunación y Bacteriología Alfonso XIII', *Dynamis*, 18, 1998, pp. 81–106.

Powell, M. 'The hidden history of social citizenship', *Citizenship Studies*, 6 (3), 2002, pp. 229–244.

Promitzer, Ch.; Trubeta, S.; Turda, M. *Health, Hygiene and Eugenics in Southeastern Europe to 1945*, Budapest: Central University Press, 2011.

Pyenson, L. 'The Ideology of Western Rationality: History of Science and the European Civilizing Mission', *Science & Education*, 2, 1993, pp. 329–343.

Pyenson, L. *Civilizing Mission: Exact Sciences and French Overseas Expansion: 1830–1940*, Baltimore: The Johns Hopkins University Press, 1993.

Pyenson, L. 'Why Science May Serve Political Ends: Cultural Imperialism and the Mission to Civilize', *Berichte zur Wissenschaftsgeschichte*, 13 (2), 1990, pp. 69–81.

Rabier, Ch. (ed.) *Fields of Expertise: A Comparative History of Expert Procedures in Paris and London, 1600 to Present*, Newcastle: Cambridge Scholars Publishing, 2007.

Raina, D. 'From West to Non-West? Basalla's Three-Stage Model Revisited', *Science as Culture*, 8 (4), 1999, pp. 497–516.

Raj, K. 'Colonial Encounters and the Forging of New Knowledge and National Identities: Great Britain and India: 1760–1850', *Osiris*, 15 (1), 2000, pp. 119–134.

Raj, K. *Relocating Modern Science: Circulation and the Construction of Knowledge in South Asia and Europe, 1650–1900*, Basingstoke: Palgrave Macmillan, 2007.

Raj, K. 'Beyond Postcolonialism and Postpositivism: Circulation and the Global History of Science', *Isis*, 104 (2), 2013, pp. 337–347.

Rees, A.M. 'The promise of social citizenship', *Policy and Politics*, 23, 1995, pp. 313–325.

Rees, A.M. (ed.) *Citizenship Today*, London: University College London Press, 1996.

Rigter, R. 'De integratie van preventieve geneeskunde in de gezondheidszorg in Nederland (1890–1940)', *Gewina*, 19, 1996, pp. 313–327.

Robert Koch-Institut des Bundesgesundheitsamtes (ed.) *100 Jahre Robert Koch-Institut*, 1. Juli 1991, Berlin: 1991.

Robert Koch-Institut (Hrsg): Gesundheit schützen, Risiken erforschen. Wer wir sind, Worauf wir zurückblicken, Was wir leisten, Berlin 2011.

Robson, W.A. *Welfare State and Welfare Society*, London: George Allen and Unwin, 1976.

Roche, M. *Rethinking Citizenship*, Cambridge: Polity Press, 1992.

Rodríguez-García, M.; Rodogno, D.; Kozma, L. (eds) *The League of Nations' Work on Social Issues*, Geneva: United Nations, 2016.

Rodríguez Ocaña, E. et al., *La acción médico-social contra el paludismo en la España metropolitana y colonial del siglo XX*, Madrid: Consejo Superior de Investigaciones Científicas, 2003.

Rosen, G. 'Economic and Social Policy in the Development of Public Health. An Essay in Interpretation', *Journal of the History of Medicine and Allied Sciences*, 8, 1953, pp. 406–430.

Rosen, G. 'Cameralism and the Concept of Medical Police', *Bulletin of the History and Medicine*, 27, 1953, pp. 21–42.

Rosen, G. 'The Fate of the Concept of Medical Police', *Centaurus*, 5, 1957, pp. 97–113.

Rosen, G. 'Mercantilism and Health Policy in Eighteenth Century French Thought', *Medical History*, 3, 1959, pp. 259–277.

Rosenberg, E.S. Spreading the American Dream: American Economic and Cultural Expansion, 1890–1945, New York: Hill & Wang, 1982.

Ruiz-Falco López, F. 'Escuela Nacional de Sanidad. Problemática pasada, actual y futura', *Revista de Sanidad e Higiene Pública*, 57, 1983, pp. 359–372.

Ryymin, T. 'Tuberculosis-threatened Children: the Rise and Fall of a Medical Concept in Norway, c. 1900-1960', *Medical History*, 52, 2008, pp. 347–364.

Said, E. *Orientalism*, London: Pantheon, 1978.

Saunier, P Y. 'Learning by Doing: Notes about the Making of the Palgrave Dictionary of Transnational History', *Journal of Modern European History*, 6, 2008, pp. 159–179.

Saunier, P.Y. *Transnational History*, Basingstoke: Palgrave Macmillan, 2013.

Schiotz, A.; Skaret, M. Det offentlige helsevesen i Norge 1603–2003. Vol II: Folkets helse-landets styrke 1850–2003, Oslo: Universiteitsforlaget, 2003.

Schultz, M.G. 'Robert Koch', *Emerging Infectious Diseases*, 17 (3), 2011, pp. 548–549.

Sealander, J. *Private Wealth and Public Life: Foundation Philanthropy and the Reshaping of American Social Policy from the Progressive Era to the New Deal*, Baltimore: The Johns Hopkins University Press, 1997.

Secord, J. 'Knowledge in Transit', *Isis*, 95, 2004, pp. 654–72.

Sigerist, H.E. 'From Bismarck to Beveridge. Developments and Trends in Social Security Legislation', *Bulletin of the History of Medicine*, 13, 1943, pp. 365–388.

Sivaramakrishnan, K. 'Global Histories of Health, Disease, and Medicine from a "Zigzag" Perspective', *Bulletin for the History of Medicine*, 89 (4) 2015, pp. 700–704.

Simonik, Peter, 'The Birth of a New System. The Rockefeller Foundation and the Institutions of the Hungarian Public Health System (1920–1935)'. In Petersen, K.; Stewart, J.; Sørensen, M.K. (eds) *American Foundations and the European Welfare States*, Odense, University of Odense, 2013, pp. 59–78.

Smith, B.H. *More than Altruism: The Politics of Private Foreign Aid*, Princeton, NJ: Princeton University Press, 1990.

Sutphen, M.P.; Bridie A. (eds) *Medicine and Colonial Identity*, London, New York: Routledge, 2003.

Swaan, A. de, *In Care of the State: Health Care, Education and Welfare in Europe and the USA in the Modern Era*, Oxford: Polity Press, 1988.

Thelen, D. 'The Nation and Beyond: Transnational Perspectives on United States History', *Journal of American History*, 8 (6), 1999, pp. 965–975.

Tournès, L. 'La philanthropie américaine, la Société des Nations et la coproduction d'un ordre international (1919–1946)', *Relations Internationales*, 151, 2012, pp. 25–36.

Trentman, F.; Just, F. (eds) *Food and Conflict in Europe in the Age of the Two World Wars*, New York: Palgrave, 2006.

Turchetti, S.; Herran, N.; Boudia, S. 'A Transnational History of Science', *British Journal for the History of Science*, 45, 2012, pp. 319–442.

Twine, F. *Citizenship and Social Rights*, London: Sage, 1994.

Tyrrell, I. 'American Exceptionalism in an Age of International History', *American Historical Review*, 96 (4), 1991, pp. 1031–1055.

Van Steenbergen, B. *The Condition of Citizenship*, London: Sage, 1994.

Vidal Hernández, J.M. *El Llatzeret de Maó, una fortalesa sanitària*, Menorca, Institut, Menorquí d'Estudis, 2002.

Vleuten, van der, E.B.A. 'Toward a transnational history of technology: meanings, promises, pitfalls', *Technology and Culture*, 49 (4), 2008, pp. 974–994.

Vogel, A. 'Who's making global civil society: Philanthropy and US empire in world society', *British Journal of Sociology*, 57 (4), 2006, pp. 636–665.

Vogel, U.; Moran. M. (ed.) *The Frontiers of Citizenship*, Basingstoke: Macmillan, 1991.

Walters, F.P. *A History of the League of Nations*, London: Oxford University Press, 1952.

Wang, Z. 'Transnational Science during the Cold War: the case of Chinese/American scientists', *Isis*, 101 (2), 2010, pp. 367–377.

Weindling, P. 'Public health and political stabilisation: The Rockefeller Foundation in central and eastern Europe between the two world wars', *Minerva*, 31, 1993, pp. 253–267.

Weindling, P. (ed.) *International Health Organisations and Movements, 1918–1939*, Cambridge: Cambridge University Press, 1995.

Weindling, P. 'Philanthropy and World Health: The Rockefeller Foundation and the League of Nations Organization', *Minerva*, 35, 1997, pp. 269–281.

Wetherby, A. The Medical Activists: Humanitarians, Activists, and American Medical Relief to Spain and China, 1936–1949, PhD Thesis, University of Oxford, 2014.

Wilkinson, L.; Hardy, A. *Prevention and Cure: The London School of Hygiene & Tropical Medicine: a 20th century quest for global public health*, London: Kegan Paul Limited, 2001.

Worboys, M. *Fractured States: Smallpox, Public Health and Vaccination Policy in British India*, Andhra Pradesh: Orient Longman, 2005.

Zunz, O. *Philanthropy in America: A History*, Princeton, New Jersey: Princeton University Press, 2011.

Zylberman, P. 'Civilizing the State: Borders, Weak States and International Health in Modern Europe', in Alison Bashford, (ed.), *Medicine at the Border: Disease, Globalization and Security, 1850 to the Present*, New York: Palgrave Macmillan, 2006, pp. 21–40.

Index

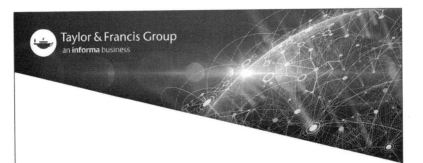

Printed and bound by CPI Group (UK) Ltd, Croydon, CR0 4YY

24/10/2024

01778282-0020